Born without Limbs

A biography of achievement

by

Kenneth Kavanagh

THE AUTHOR

Kenneth Kavanagh was born in Staffordshire and taught in schools in France before joining the Probation Service in England. He is currently Senior Divorce Court Welfare Officer in Bedfordshire, and also serves on the Parliamentary all-party Family and Child Protection Group at Westminster.

He is married and has four children.

© K H Kavanagh, 1989

Published by
Family Publications
Wicken, Milton Keynes, MK19 6BU
Tel: 0908 57234

Cover design by the Benedictines at Turvey Abbey

Printed in Great Britain by
BPCC Wheatons Ltd
Marsh Barton, Exeter, EX2 8RP

ISBN 1 871217 03 2

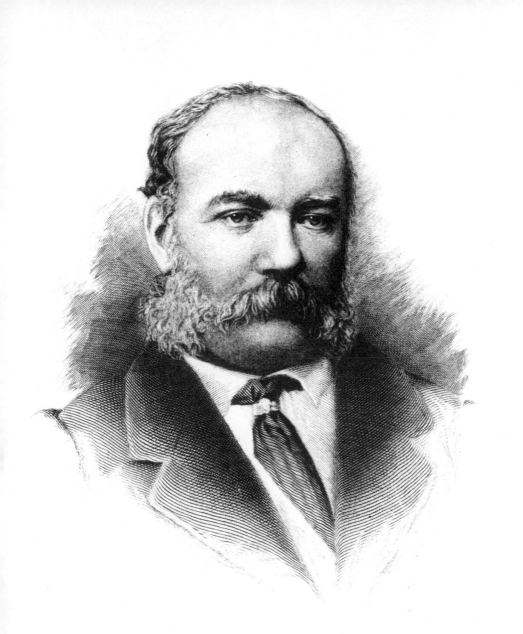

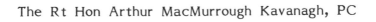
The Rt Hon Arthur MacMurrough Kavanagh, PC

CONTENTS

AUTHOR'S NOTE

Arthur MacMurrough Kavanagh was one of the most remarkable figures of the 19th century. He was a grandson of the seventeenth Earl of Ormonde, one of the richest Irish landowners, and of the second Earl of Clancarty, one of the most skilful diplomatists of the period. Although he was born without arms or legs, he became an accomplished traveller and sportsman, a Member of Parliament at Westminster and a Privy Councillor.

Although my common ancestry with Arthur Kavanagh is too remote to be of any consequence, his legendary figure has interested me since childhood, as a man who achieved the seemingly impossible. This interest was revived recently while exploring the neglected little chapel in the ancient Kavanagh burial ground at St Mullins, where his mother, Lady Harriet Kavanagh, who was a powerful influence on his development, is buried.

Arthur Kavanagh died one hundred years ago, and this short biography is intended to mark that event. In writing it I am indebted to Mr and Mrs Andrew MacMurrough Kavanagh for giving me access to the originals of the Kavanagh papers at Borris House and for sharing recollections and anecdotes with me; to The Hon Desmond Guinness for allowing me access to the unpublished letters of Lady Louisa Conolly, the property of the Castletown Foundation, and to Mrs Lena Boylan for her work on those letters; to Mrs Boylan and Mrs Annette Camier, Principal of Celbridge National School for helping me to identify places associated with Arthur Kavanagh's childhood. I am also indebted to Mr C Fahy, Assistant Keeper of the National Library of Ireland for his guidance in working on the Kavanagh papers housed in the Library; to Miss Aideen Ireland, Archivist at the Public Records Office, Dublin; to Mrs Coleman of the Land Registry,

Henrietta Street, Dublin; to Mary Kavanagh and Eileen
Farragher of the Galway County Library Services; to
Margaret Phelan and Frank Kavanagh of the Kilkenny
Archaeological Society; to P J Kavanagh for guiding
me through the Irish Press of the 19th century; and to
Carmel Flahavan of Carlow County Library for providing
me with local source material.

I am also indebted to Sir Trevor Street, MP, to Betty
McInnes of the House of Commons Library; to the Clerk
of Records, House of Lords Records Office, who provided
the specimens of Arthur Kavanagh's handwriting from the
Ashbourne papers; and to the staff of the British Library
for identifying material relating to Arthur Kavanagh in
the Gladstone papers.

Where I have had difficulty in transcribing letters in
the Kavanagh Papers, particularly those of Lady Harriet
because of her habit of writing both horizontally and
vertically on the paper, I have drawn on the existing
transcriptions of Sarah Steele and Donald McCormick
with appropriate acknowledgements.

I am grateful to the Rev John O'Leary of Paulstown, Co
Kilkenny, to Kathleen O'Shea of Drumgriffin, Co Galway;
to Sister Philomena of the Sisters of Mercy at Callan,
to the Sisters of Mercy at Ballyragget Lodge, and to
Betty Young of Old Lorum for their recollections of
local lore on Arthur Kavanagh. I am also indebted to
the staff of the North Bedfordshire Library for their
patient assistance with background material, to Mr John
Bennet for deciphering my handwriting, and to my wife
for her encouragement and the sketch of Borris House.

Kenneth H Kavanagh
Bedford, August 1989

FOREWORD

This is the story of a baby born over a hundred years ago.

The birth of Arthur Kavanagh, the third son of an Irish Landlord, was surrounded with superstition when it was known that he had no limbs.

Had this biography been about overcoming disability in present day times, it would have been interesting; but Arthur was born in 1831, which makes his adventures even more remarkable. The book combines biography with history, including the problems of the Irish potato famine; it showed how easy it was for Arthur's mother, Lady Harriet, to escape to foreign parts because she had the means to do so.

Because Arthur had determination and backing, he was able to travel the world before settling down in Ireland to family life. When he was in India and had become short of funds, he was described by one of his compatriots as "a wonderful horseman, he spent most of his time riding, though he could hop about on his stumps with astonishing agility. He made great friends with the native children and often used to sit under a tree in the garden, painting them as they sat in wonderment at this surprising man who held a brush so dextrously between his two stumps."

When back in Ireland, he became a Magistrate and a Member of Parliament at Westminster.

It is a book which I am sure will give encouragement to many people who read it, as it shows what can be done with determination and will power.

Baroness Masham of Ilton

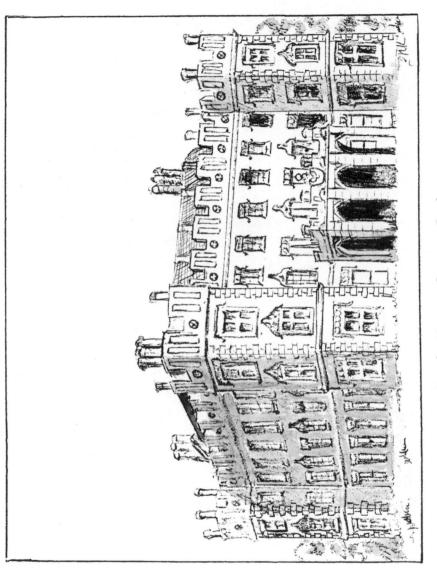

Borris House, County Carlow

1. A SON IS BORN . . .

Thomas Kavanagh, gentleman, soldier, landlord, apostate, boasted an impeccable Celtic-Irish descent. Athletic and virile, he had a capacity for producing daughters. By his marriage to Lady Elizabeth Butler, daughter of the 17th Earl of Ormonde, he had nine and one ailing son. By his marriage to Lady Harriet le Poer Trench, daughter of the 2nd Earl of Clancarty, he had one daughter and two sons. When Lady Harriet became pregnant again in the summer of 1830 Thomas, then sixty four and as old as his wife's father, gladly accepted a wager of a bottle of claret from the family physician Francis Boxwell, that the child to be born soon after St Patrick's Day the following year, would be a boy.

The birth took place on the 25th of March, the Feast of the Annunciation of the Blessed Virgin Mary, in both the calendar of the Catholic Church which Thomas had deserted and the Church of Ireland to which he had conformed. Before the sun rose over the Blackstairs Mountains or the birds stirred in the woods around Borris House, the Kavanagh home in County Carlow, Francis Boxwell knew he had won his wager. It gave him no joy; there was no relish in claiming his prize. The child he had delivered was a strong healthy boy with, "a nobly proportioned head and trunk," but without arms or legs.(1) At dawn a nurse wrapped the new born child in red flannel and sat rocking him in dismay. Boxwell told Thomas and Thomas told Lady Harriet. It was a day of mixed feelings. By evening, when Lady Harriet's candles burned low and the embers glowed in the fire-places of Borris House, neither miracle nor death had solved the problem. The child slept, his truncated limbs covered by his gown; on seeing him for the first time his mother enigmatically thanked God that he was born to her and no one else.

The child's ancestry was fascinating. The Kavanaghs of Borris were "the oldest family in the British Empire," (2) tracing their descent in legend from Fenusius of Scythia, through the early kings of Ireland to the present time. They were in the main tough and turbulent-warrior horse-men but in the 7th century had produced their own saint, Moling, Bishop of Ferns, who founded a monastery just down river from Borris where many of them lay in peace in its ruins after a life-time of violent conflict.

Lady Harriet was descended, through her mother from a Donegal publican and the beheaded Earl of Strafford. The le Poer Trenches, her father's family, were acquisitive and ambitious; their political star was rising. Neither family had a history of tolerance for the weak and vulnerable.

A simplistic version of Irish history attributes the emnity and divisions which have plagued Ireland for a thousand years to two men fighting over one woman. In 1167, having abducted the daughter of the King of Connacht and fearing revenge, Dermot MacMurrough invited the Earl of Pembroke into Ireland to assist him. With his superior forces Pembroke subdued Dermot's enemies, married his daughter and claimed his succession as King of Leinster. It was to curb the growing power of Pembroke, otherwise known as Strongbow, that Henry II intervened and established an English interest in the business of Ireland. From Dermot's son, surnamed Kavanagh after the place of his upbringing, Kilcavan in County Wicklow, sprang a race of warrior-kings who dominated the Province of Leinster for the next two hundred years and who were in the forefront of the endless wars to oust the English. In the fourteenth century Art MacMurrough Kavanagh, "at whose puisance all Leinster trembled,"(3) was one of those "rough rug-headed kerns" of Shakespeare's Richard II who harassed the English from hide-outs in the mountains and forests of Carlow and Wexford. He was great of stature, rode without a saddle a horse worth two hundred cows, and galloped like the wind. Subdued by Richard II, he was knighted and then rose again in rebellion which lasted until his death.

For officers of the English crown, freedom of passage was not assured in 'Kavanagh Country' until the reign of Henry VIII, when the Kavanagh's at last did homage and were recognized as 'chieftains' in return. Even at that time they mustered as many cavalry as the king in Leinster.

The Kavanaghs continued in an ambivalent relationship with the English crown, sometimes conforming, sometimes in revolt. Morgan, brought up in England with his brother and two sisters settled his estates in 1621, and styled himself 'Kavanagh of Borris', having acquired the lands forfeited by the less pliant Ryans.(4) His son Bryan, as a Protestant, escaped the Cromwellian confiscations while others of the Kavanagh clan chose exile rather than conformity. The senior branch of the clan, dispossessed of their fertile acres around Castletown in North Carlow, were transplanted to less hospitable terrain west of the Shannon on the shores of Loch Corrib in 1655. Others chose exile in Europe and resurfaced in the eighteenth century as chamberlains at the court of the Empress Maria Teresa. Charles Kavanagh was Governor of Prague in 1766 and Joseph Kavanagh was in the forefront of the assault on the Bastille.

A hundred years after Morgan settled at Borris the Kavanaghs were Catholic again and despite the penal laws, amassing land through dynastic marriages with the family of the Earls of Ormonde, whose annual income exceeded that of many a German prince. Thomas Kavanagh's paternal grandmother was the sister of the 15th Earl, his mother was the daughter of the 16th Earl, and his first wife the daughter of the 17th Earl.

The penal laws following the victory of William III over James II excluded Catholics from Parliament, from office under the crown, from the armed forces and the professions and made inheritance uncertain when the law was rigorously enforced. It was not unusual for the heir to ar. estate to conform outwardly to Protestantism to retain his lands while the rest of the family remained Catholic. Thomas' father was a signatory of the petition for the Relief of Catholics. Thomas himself, a second son, was brought up in the Catholic Faith and inherited his lands at Ballyragget in Kilkenny from his cousin Robert Butler for that reason, but "ere Robert Butler was ten years in his grave Thomas, the representative of one of the most Catholic Houses in Ireland, had gone over to Protestantism, and been elected to the Irish Parliament."(5)

In a romantic interlude in Thomas' youth his aunt, Lady Eleanor Butler - one of the Ladies of Llangollen - had been imprisoned in Borris House after an unsuccessful flight from Kilkenny Castle to elope with her friend Sarah Ponsonby.

The American declaration of Independence had stirred Irish Protestants dissatisfied with the degree of English involvement in Irish affairs, and the French Revolution had sown seeds of Republicanism. The United Irishmen, a radical movement seeking Parliamentary reform and the union of Catholic and Protestant in Ireland, made little headway and by 1796 had become a secret society dedic-ated to bringing change through violence. They invited the revolutionary French into Ireland to help them break the English connection and in December of that year thirty five ships sailed into Bantry Bay. Drawn up on shore was a meagre force of militia-men commanded by William Trench, Lady Harriet's grandfather, hoping to appear as the vanguard of a larger, but in reality non-existent force. Sleet, snow and storms prevented the French from landing and gales eventually blew the ships back out to the Atlantic. Although the weather defeated the would-be-invaders, William Trench was rewarded for his presence with a seat in the Irish House of Lords, as Baron Kilconnel.

Ruthless repression followed the failure of the invading forces at Bantry. Brutal flogging and capping with burning pitch were commonplace until the Irish, led in some instances by their priests, rose in rebellion in 1798. Borris House was besieged by insurgents who were repulsed by Thomas Kavanagh at the head of the local militia. Although the rebellion collapsed, the

British Government was forced to face up to the Irish Question. Protestants now thought of maintaining their ascendancy in association with Protestant England, though some of them opposed union of the two Parliaments on the grounds that it would mean the end of the Kingdom of Ireland established by Henry VIII in 1534. Some Catholics favoured such a union because they believed, it offered them the protection of a more tolerant English Protestant majority. Richard Trench, Lady Harriet's father voted against the union of the Dublin and Westminster Parliaments in 1799 but in 1800 having been "squared" by Castlereagh, one of his wife's kinsmen, with the promise of an Earldom for his father, he voted for it.(6) On January the first 1801 the Irish Parliament was abolished and the two kingdoms united "forever". Thomas Kavanagh, who had represented Kilkenny since 1798, was among those who lost their seats.

"The noble family of Trench," as Lady Harriet's father described them, were Huguenot merchants who fled from France after the massacre of Saint Bartholomew.(7) They made their way to England and then to Ireland where they acquired extensive lands during the Cromwellian upheavals. They claimed an important role in William of Orange's victory over the Catholic Irish having exposed a Jacobite plot and acted as guides to the king. In fifty years they "rose from humble origins to a position of great wealth."(8) The marriage of Richard Trench to Francis Power in 1732 gave them a slender connection with the Norman knight Geoffre le Poer and the ancient Earls of Clancarty, and they adopted the name le Poer Trench.

Lady Hariet's father, born in 1767, was educated at Newcomes Academy, a school in Hackney "for gentlemen and the sons of nobility" where swearing was "inveterate". (9) After studying at St. John's College Cambridge and Lincolns Inn he was called to the Bar in Ireland in 1793 and in 1796 married Harriet Staples, the daughter of Judge John Staples, a man considered "vulgar" and "in the common run" by his wife's family.(10)

In 1803 the le Poer Trenches were rewarded for their support of Pitt in his stratagems to bring about the Union of Ireland and England, with the revival in their favour, of the ancient Earldom of Clancarty. Lady Harriet's father succeeded to the title in 1805 and his rise was rapid. He became Master of the Mint, Post Master General, Commissioner for India and a Senior Plenipotentiary at the Congress of Vienna in the absence of the Duke of Wellington. Tallyrand wrote to Louis XVIII of Clancarty's "zeal, firmness and uprightness."(11) He negotiated the abortive arrangements for the marriage of the Prince of Orange to the princess Charlotte, daughter of George IV, and facilitated plans for the union of the Dutch and Belgian provinces into the new Kingdom of the Netherlands. When the Prince of Orange became King he accompanied him to the Hague as British Ambassador, where he remained until 1823. When he left he was rewarded with the title Marquis of Heusden. Wellington regarded him as a model landlord "who visited his estates in Ireland instead of bawling and brawling in London."(12) He kept Wellington informed on the state of Ireland and in 1827 Wellington tipped him as a possible successor to Lord Liverpool as Prime Minister.

Clancarty was a man of ability, energy and determination; "a bustling hard man;" a good lawyer, a kind man to his family but above all a thorough manager of his estates.(13) The town of Balinasloe, adjacent to his seat in County Galway, was transformed under his influence and that of his family, from a slum with impassable streets and dung piled high as the eaves, into a pleasant place with wide thoroughfares. Canals were cut and later on railways were built; fairs and markets were sited and entertainments organised for the tenants who were ruled with "a wreath or rod." Ale houses closed at "a reasonable hour," vagabonds and "idle women" were sent to the Bridewell and no one dared throw down even a bowl of water.(14)

Lord Clancarty's brother Power rose with equal rapidity within the Church of Ireland becoming first Bishop of Waterford, then Bishop of Elphin and finally, in 1819,

Archbishop of Tuam. His preferment was attributed as much to his lavish entertainment of the Viceroy, the Duke of Richmond, as to his ability; he managed to combine his episcopal responsibilities with a captaincy in the yeomanry, scouring the countryside at night for rebels.

The Weslyans had preached in the West of Ireland in the previous century and the le Poer Trenches, carried along in a post-Weslyan tide of evangelical zeal, identified themselves with the proselytising activities of the Hibernian Bible Society for whom "the most legitimate field of labour . . . is in the professed region of Popery, where there are few or no Protestants to show the deluded multitude a more excellent way."(15) On their estates in Connacht in furtherance of these aims, the le Poer Trenches set up neat thatched Bible Schools where Catholic children were taught the Protestant catechism encouraged in their learning by material rewards. At one stage they were accused, not without some justification, of diverting public money intended for the development of Catholic schools into their own Bible Schools; their activities destroyed the feelings of mutual acceptance which had been developing between the Catholic and Protestant clergy for over fifty years. The response of the Catholic clergy in Balinasloe to the distribution of Protestant Bibles, which they considered erroneous, was to collect them and throw them in the river.

In March 1824 Lady Granville wrote a double-edged description of Lady Clancarty, Lady Harriet's mother; and of Lady Harriet, her sister Louisa and their brother. Lady Clancarty, Lady Granville wrote, "is an excellent, head aching woman but without the insolent manners of the wife of an ambassador and with two ugly and obliging daughters and a ditto son."(16)

In February 1825 Lady Harriet, "ugly and obliging," married Thomas Kavanagh. For Thomas, approaching sixty and with ten children; and for Harriet, twenty five, unattractive and with antecedents which noted a streak of the vulgar and a "very small share" of sense, it was probably the best match either could have hoped for.(17)

When Lady Harriet arrived at Borris, a house in the Italian and Lombard style, set in some of the most beautiful scenery in Ireland, her family and admirers saw her as the perfect wife, the perfect mother for Thomas' children and the perfect mistress of the great house, who would quickly endear herself to the tenants. Others saw her as the suspect daughter of a proselytising "union peer" - enobled for his role in the destruction of the Irish Parliament and who, it was wrongly assumed, had weaned her aging suitor from the Catholic religion as the price of marriage. She was a "parvenue", the pleasure seeking daughter of a second Earl who had filched the styles and titles of the ancient Earldom of Clancarty; an unworthy successor to the aristocratic Lady Elizabeth; and although her family had been in Ireland for a hundred and fifty years, they were still regarded as aliens.

2. INFANCY

On Christmas Eve 1830 Francis Boxwell rode to Borris
House with presents for Lady Harriet's children; young
Harriet aged five, Tom four and Charlie two. Boxwell had
studied medicine in Glasgow and Dublin, was in charge
of the dispensaries at Borris and Glynn, was medical
attendant at the local fever hospital and physician to
the local constabulary. Lady Harriet, who was six months
pregnant, liked him, had confidence in him and enjoyed
his visits. "His rare invigorating smile, so unprofessional,"
she described as being "like a ray of sunshine from
heaven." In turn Boxwell admired her patience and
cheerfulness. She was healthy, determined and, in his
view, too active for her condition. He had a hunch that
this latest pregnancy might bring problems. There was
"a definite weakness" from an earlier pregnancy; "some
displacement"; "but nothing to trouble the patient."[1]
He was convinced she was riding too much and forbade
it. Throughout the pregnancy she took, with or without
Boxwell's approval, a "herbal remedy."[2]

Whether or not Boxwell's attendant screamed in horror,
as folk-lore alleges, when the child was delivered, is
a matter for conjecture; but the doctor was tormented
by the thought that with greater foresight and skill he
might have prevented the deformities. He believed, with
respectable medical opinion of the time, that "by an
intra-uterine complication well nigh unique in the annals
of gynaecology the umbilical cord constricting and
amputating legs and arms alike, just below the upper
third," had resulted in the child being "brought into the
world with all the disadvantages incident to defective
means of locomotion and prehension."[3] It was a view
that persisted in medical circles for more than half a
century.

A range of the concerned and unconcerned throughout
Carlow and Kilkenny speculated, each according to his or
her own prejudices, on the causes of the strange birth.

The kinder local gossips attributed the deformities to the unknown herbal remedy, while in Kilkenny it was said that Lady Harriet had refused alms to a beggar who had cursed the child in her womb. Some saw the hand of God at work. "Catholic scullery maids at Borris had brought a small statue of the Virgin and Child into the kitchen from a local mission. Lady Harriet finding it there threw it to the floor in a fit of Protestant zeal, smashing it. When the pieces were gathered up, the arms and legs of the infant Christ were missing."(4) It was too great a coincidence that when her son was born on the Feast of the Annunciation of the Blessed Virgin, marking the visit of the Angel Gabriel to Mary telling her she was to be the mother of the Messiah, he was without arms or legs.

The Kavanaghs of Borris believe that when the statues of the Blessed Virgin and St Joseph were removed from the family chapel in Borris House on its re-ordering for Protestant worship, they were accidentally damaged by workmen; this took on a special significance after 1831.

The less pious turned to the 'Legend of the Cripple' for an explanation. The Kavanaghs who had invited the Normans into Ireland with all the ensuing strife and misery would, it was said, be cursed until the heir was a cripple. A local woman receiving rough justice from Thomas Kavanagh had renewed the curse, prophesying that when the withered branch of the oak tree in the courtyard at Borris fell, a crippled child would be born. The withered branch fell in 1830 and the "crippled child" was born the following year but he was not the heir; not yet at least.

At the time of the strange birth Thomas' heir, Walter, was sixteen; six of Thomas' daughters remained unmarried. Mary had married and was dead before she was fourteen and was buried at St Mullins. Agnes the youngest fitted well with Lady Harriet's three older children. When this little group peered into their new-born brother's cradle they saw a baby "with beautiful intelligent eyes, a broad brow and a clear fair skin." Like most babies he gave them "a grave look" or "broke into smiles."(5) They did notice the sleeves of his gown tied up like small bags but were unaware of his handicaps.

Dr Boxwell concluded that this child could not be locked away in an isolated room like Thomas, the monster son of the Earl of Strathmore, seen only by servants and allowed exercise at night. Calling the staff together in Borris House he talked about the new born child and with tongue in cheek took up the story of the Kavanagh's curse. Nature was inscrutable like Providence, he said, and if she had robbed the child of arms and legs she would give him other and more valuable assets. "I tried," he later wrote, "to show them the legend in a different light; to seize on the point in it which seemed to me practical and sensible when dealing with such people - to wit the idea that this could be the turning point in a whole community's fortunes and co-incidentally in their own lives as villagers and tenants of the Kavanaghs. The boy, I said, would make good and confound them although at the time I hardly dared accept my own optimism."(6) Lady Harriet's niece, Sarah Steel wrote, "From the outset it was manifest that his upbringing must be different from that of other men for he was without limbs . . ."(7) Boxwell took a different view. He proposed, and Lady Harriet accepted, that the child's education should be their joint project and he set out his plans in a letter to her:

"I have not forgotten you and your boy (Art) on this visit to Dublin. I talked to Dr Marsh and various specialists who believe in due course some mechanical means of propulsion can be provided for him. You have displayed wondrous patience and cheerfulness over all this and I never cease to marvel at it. Our joint task must be to make (him) entirely unconscious of his limitations, or his disabilities, as far as is humanly possible.

"This I do assure you, is far easier for one born as he is than it would be for a grown up boy who had suddenly lost his limbs. Therefore I say that because of this our battle is already half won. We

must make him unaware of fear from the cradle.
It may seem cruel to appear indifferent, to ignore
his screams and not let him feel dependent on you
but in the end it will be an immense kindness.
If he has no fears, he will not hesitate to take
risks and risks he must eventually take if he is to
become as other children.

"But above all he must be made conscious of his
heritage and instilled with a sense of destiny. He
must feel in his bones that he has a mission to
fulfill, for this is the only way in which he will
overcome his grievous handicap. But again he is
fortunate in having a family who by their manifold
examples, can point the way for him."(6)

By the choice of a name the boy was made conscious
of his heritage - Arthur MacMurrough Kavanagh, after
his 14th century ancestor, the warrior horseman who
"galloped like the wind" and "at whose puissance all
Leinster trembled."(6)

Lady Harriet believed that while adversity was the will
of God and to be accepted, it was intended to refine
and not to crush. In her regular Bible readings she found
numerous examples of the human spirit rising above
difficulties. If she prayed as though all depended on
God, she acted as though all depended on her energy,
determination and a good use of resources. She was
her father's daughter. Boxwell encouraged her, praising
her good humour, flattering her and with a touch of
the Blarney invited her to believe that Arthur would
have treble the strength in his brain and body because
it would not be dissipated through his arms and legs.
There was, at last, enthusiasm in Borris House for
Arthur's future while outside suspicion and superstitions
remained.

The birth of "a monster" to the proselytising Earl of
Clancarty's iconoclastic daughter confirmed to many
local people that, like her father, she was evil. When
her carriage again drove out of the crenallated gateway,

"the warning passed down the village that Lady Harriet
was coming in her phaeton and everybody ran in doors;
she was considered by the locals to be such an evil
person."(10)   She returned to her former lifestyle considered brave by her friends and brazen by her enemies.
Her decision to build a chapel at Ballyragget, which she
refused to have consecrated and which she offered instead
to anyone with anything good to say was to her traducers
disturbing defiance of custom.

Arthur grew in the care of his nurse Anne Flemming.
All the usual demands made of a child were made of him
and the customary frustrations were used as stimuli. Anne
would place his toys just out of reach and encourage him
to wriggle towards them.   Where other children grasped
them clumsily in their hands Arthur grasped them between
his small stumps and learned to flick them in a swift
scissor movement. Once he could sit up he quickly learned
to propel himself across the room by bouncing.

His aunt Lady Louisa le Poer Trench saw him as " the
most handsome of all the children, and not withstanding
that the use of the word may seem faintly ridiculous
when applied to one so young, he has a 'noble' mien."
He had "quite the noblest head in the family."(11)
"All who received the little boy badly on the day of
his birth," says Mary McCarthy, "had now begun to
love him."(12)

By 1833 Arthur was often seen by the villagers, a
handsome fair haired little boy strapped firmly, in
the saddle in front of Boxwell.   From Boxwells's horse
he first saw the old deer park, the great beech trees,
the banks of rhododendrons and the thick woods which
surrounded the house.   Together they watched the birds
and the squirrels and listened to the waters of the brook
rushing down towards the Barrow and the sea.

"God has blessed man with the horse", the doctor wrote,
"for Art Kavanagh the horse will be the greatest blessing
of all. I have urged that as soon as he is old enough to
sit upright, he should be given a pony and strapped to it.

There is no need for fear as to his safety. He will survive accidents for he is tough and wiry."(13)

On his fourth birthday Lady Harriet gave Arthur a pony and, strapped into a basket saddle, he was led by his brothers around the estate. In the same year he learned to propel himself through the house and out to the stables in a mechanical chair. To less accessible places he was carried by a servant.

Lady Harriet spent her time sketching and painting the splendid views around Borris. Mount Leinster and the Blackstairs Mountains rose above woodlands and the golden fields of summer corn. Arthur often sat watching his mother until one day she drew a triangle on her pad, placed the brush between his teeth and invited him to copy it. She writes with pride in her diary, "I painted a simple triangle and urged Arthur to try it. He looked quite incredulous that I should think him capable of such a feat, but after several attempts he succeeded in making a recognizable, if somewhat crude, copy of what I had set him to do."(14)

Arthur's first five years were like those of many children, years of discovery and enchantment. For his father they were years of turmoil and decline. Thomas' response to the birth had been one of bitterness and shame. He had been athletic in his youth and was now a laughing stock to his enemies. Some of his contemporaries regarded him, since his conforming to Protestantism over thirty years earlier, as "the last chieftain and first heretic of his race," (15) strangely punished for his desertion of the Catholic religion by his son's deformities. Within months of the birth, Thomas found himself politically out manoeuvred.

The Union of the Dublin and Westminster Parliaments in 1801 had cost Thomas his seat as MP for Kilkenny, and Ireland its Parliament. The promised prosperity and reconciliation had not been brought about. Thomas had not re-entered Parliament until 1826, the year following his marriage to Lady Harriet when he was returned unopposed in Carlow.

Catholic emancipation had been achieved only after twenty nine years of agitation. In the process Daniel O'Connel, the Catholic barrister from Kerry, forged a movement uniting peasantry, the middle classes and the Catholic clergy, which threatened the positions of landlords even in County Carlow. Demands for the advancement of Catholics in government were no problem for Thomas, brought up in that faith and with his sister Honora, a nun in an English convent; but an increase in the influence and power of the 'lower orders' threatened his position as a landlord and that was unacceptable.

In the election campaign following the death of George IV, the O'Connelites and Liberals gained such support that Thomas and his son-in-law Henry Bruen withdrew from the contest rather than risk defeat. In 1832 both stood again and were defeated. During that campaign the Carlow Morning Post published an article on Thomas' conforming to Protestantism; it was judged defamatory and brought him damages of fifteen hundred pounds.

The election campaign of 1835 proved a very bitter one. Thomas addressed the voters through the columns of the Carlow Sentinel and Kilkenny Advertiser. "With the security and self possession of his class he proposed no definite programme merely mentioning his former record which he did not elaborate on, as sufficient reason for voters to support him."(16)   The Kilkenny Moderator urged readers to vote for him as "the scion of the oldest family in the British Empire and possessed of a princely income, a large portion of which is spent in improving the condition and promoting the comforts of his poorer neighbours."

In Borris he was opposed by the Catholic clergy - Father John Walshe senior, parish priest and John Walshe junior, his curate and nephew. When John Walshe senior addressed the Kavanagh tenants at Glynn, Thomas arrived with the militia and took his tenants back to Borris to be "cooped" under his protection until they had voted as he wished. When Father Walshe junior was found dead at Kilgranny bridge the landlords were accused of killing him, though he seems to have died when he fell, accidentally, from his horse. Thomas was further accused and cleared of partiality in his judgements as a magistrate.

The validity of the 1835 election, which returned Thomas and Henry to Westminster, was challenged on the grounds that their agents obstructed O'Connelite voters from reaching the polling booths in time to vote by administering separate oaths against bribery and on property qualifications to each elector. Fresh elections were ordered in which Thomas was defeated. Both he and Henry Bruen petitioned on the grounds that a number of their opponents were of insufficient substance to qualify for the vote. The petition was upheld and Thomas and Henry declared elected. Agitation in the area became so great that Thomas, fearing an attack on Borris House, wrote twice to Dublin requesting troops be sent to protect him.

Thomas was now seventy. The turbulent campaign had reached its lowest point with the pinning of references to the "cripple Kavanagh" on the chapel door in Bagnalstown, and had destroyed his health. His heir Walter died suddenly in 1836 and Thomas himself died in January 1837, "from the effects of gout that had reached his stomach."(17)

The Carlow Sentinel, uncritical of the landlord class, wrote "On Tuesday morning last, the remains of the much revered and respected gentleman were conveyed from Borris House to the family vaults in St Mullins amidst cries and lamentations of hundreds of the poor peasantry and their families who lived upon his bounty for years. So heart-rending a scene was never witnessed as the hearse passing through the gates into the town of Borris." He had been a man of few words, "a most kind and indulgent landlord;" a defender of the political and social status quo, "high minded," "an impartial magistrate," possessed of a "princely fortune" and "descended from a princely race," who had "fed the hungry and clothed the naked." According to The Sentinel, the funeral procession was two miles long and joined by workers leaving the fields, as tributaries swelling a stream, until ten thousand gathered around the grave, "uttering curses both loud and deep on the heartless miscreant who would dare insult the most kind hearted and honourable man the century has ever produced." The scene is somewhat exaggerated, for the tiny chapel at St Mullins in which Thomas was buried could accommodate no more than one hundred persons.

The "heartless miscreant" was O'Connel, who said to a crowd in Carlow, "Poor Kavanagh! Alas Poor Kavanagh. If he had not made a disgraceful connection he would have died in peace and not have the cats and dogs of the neighbourhood thrust into his grave with him."(18)

3.   A CHILD DESERTED

Following her husband's death, Lady Harriet went to Torquay on the pretext of finding a school for her step daughter Agnes, and showed little interest in returning. Tom, heir to the Borris Estates, was nine and unable to succeed for another twelve years. Arthur, now six, enjoyed the journey to Torquay and liked the place.

The Kavanagh tenants, who had wept around Thomas' grave, found "the patron of the poor," replaced by the hard headed tight-fisted Earl of Clancarty, as the administrator of the Estates. Clancarty had definite views on the need for reorganisation and economies, usually at the expense of the tenants, and Doyne, Thomas' agent, was a willing collaborator.

On St Patrick's Day Lord Clancarty wrote to Doyne, "I must fully agree with you upon the necessity of diminishing the expenditure of Borris, as early and as much as may be practicable. Your kind and able advice will scarcely fail of being my principal, I might say my only guide upon this important matter."(1)

Outgoing tenants could expect no favours and those in difficulty no help, except encouragement to emigrate, though Clancarty assured Doyne that he was not an advocate of emigration except as a means of getting rid of "obnoxious characters."

Perusing the accounts he noted a claim by one of the Kavanaghs' man-servants for £10 for the cost of a journey to London and would, he said, certainly have paid it had it been his own money he was administering. However, he could not help noting that his own son travelled the greater distance from Garbally to London for six guineas and he thought that was a far more appropriate sum. He was less inclined to challenge the accounts of Mrs Wax, one of Lady Harriet's servants, whom he found "not one of the most gentle of her sex."

Her account was settled in full as Lady Harriet regarded her as "a domestic, valuable and intelligent."(2)

Clancarty was irritated by his daughter's continuing absence which he found "untoward," and a hindrance to his plans. She fared little better than the tenants and neither sentiment nor the need for her comfort influenced him. He wanted her to reside permanently at Borris as the best means of preventing dilapidations, keeping the house aired and preserving the paintings. Her "regrettable," absence prevented him from disposing of the "extra" furniture, but he ordered Doyne to draw up inventories and proceed with valuations in preparation for a public sale of the contents of the house. Lady Harriet could, if she wished, "purchase any items of furniture for her future convenience."(3)

Always seeking to be seen as a fair man Clancarty, as an executer of Thomas' will, took pains to ensure that Thomas' daughters by his first marriage, who inherited under the will of their grandmother the Countess of Ormonde, were protected. He was zealous in reminding Doyne, however, that Thomas had shown equal solicitude for the children of his second marriage and his own grandchildren, and that in the final distribution "all should receive equal shares."(4)

When Lady Harriet returned to Borris her father and Doyne presented her with their long discussed plans. She was to take "the whole concern" into her occupation, and under her "superintendency." This included the house, gardens, shrubberies, offices, plantations and "other lands," plus sixty acres in the deer park and two hundred acres in the demesne. The latter was to be let out during Tom's minority thus avoiding the expense of stewarding and labourers' wages.(5) She accepted Borris House as her principal residence but in the following November her father died and she was finally free to indulge her passion for prolonged periods of travel abroad, leaving the Estate in the hands of Doyne.

She was an enthusiastic European, having spent much

of her youth at the Dutch Court while her father
was ambassador there. With his involvement in the
negotiations for the marriage of Princess Charlotte
and in the deliberations of the Congress of Vienna, she
had lived on the exciting fringes of history. At fifteen
she danced at "the most famous ball in history" given
by the Duchess of Richmond at her house in the rue
de la Blanchiserie in Brussels on the eve of Waterloo,
and her father gave her pearls for the occasion. It
was a glittering night of Princes, aristocrats, generals
and their ladies. Though the restored Napoleon and
his forces were not far away, a nonchalant Wellington
reminisced with the revellers about life in Ireland and
early morning rides in Phoenix Park. When the Prince
of Orange brought news of Napoleon's thrust towards
Quatre Bras the mood changed; officers said goodbye to
their ladies and then hurried out into the warm evening
to join the red and green and blue-jacketed soldiers
leaving the city, many to die and many to return
maimed. Back in the ballroom Lady Georgina Lennox
was shocked to find "some energetic and heartless
young ladies still dancing." Lady Harriet's subsequent
detractors liked to think she was one of them. Later
that evening the revellers listened to the sounds of
the distant battle from the city ramparts.

Marriage and child bearing had curtailed Lady Harriet's
travels; but now a widow and rich, Borris, however
beautiful, could not hold her.

With Tom and Charley at Eton and Arthur painstakingly
busy learning to write with a pen in his mouth or held
tight between his stumps in the schoolroom at Borris,
Lady Harriet returned to her favourite haunts in Paris,
Florence, Rome and Corfu, coming back from time to
time to show the sketches and paintings she made as
records of her journeys. Arthur kept in touch with her
through laboriously written notes on small squares of
blue paper with carefully ruled lines. "Melford says
'I'm a very good boy, and I send you a kiss.'" There
were occasional hints of sadness in "I wish Hoddy (his
sister) was here to ride with me on Battle."(6)

When Arthur was eight his mother sent him to live at Celbridge in County Kildare. It is a small village on the banks of the Liffey, twelve miles from Dublin. The main street broadens into an avenue of limes, and in autumn a carpet of brown and gold leaves stretches to a point where the eye can see no further. Walking under the trees makes the avenue seem shorter and suddenly, not in front but to one side, is one of Ireland's most magnificent houses. "An Italian town palace of Farnese proportions," built in silver limestone, it stretches its colonnaded arms around a garden of yews.(7) In the eighteenth and nineteenth centuries this was Castletown, the home of Lady Harriet's Conolly cousins. Built by Galilei in 1722 for William Conolly, son of a Ballyshannon publican, who became speaker of the Irish House of Commons and who made his fortune dealing in the for- feited estates of others, it was a model of eighteenth century elegance with walls hung with green silk, and galleries lit by Venetian chandeliers. Above and around its splendid staircase by the Dutch-Italian Vierpyl, clusters of cherubs hung in breathtaking splendour. The large crack in the elegant mirror in the dining room was said to have been caused by a priestly encounter with the devil. Speaker Conolly returning one day from hunting with a guest, noticed a cloven hoof when the guest removed his boots. When he refused to leave, Speaker Conolly sent for the priest. The Devil was unimpressed by the rite of exorcism and the frustrated priest threw the book at him; the Devil sidestepped and the book hit the mirror.

Lady Harriet's mother grew up at Castletown. She was a granddaughter of the beheaded Earl of Strafford and the daughter of Judge John Staples, a man considered vulgar by the Conollys. Little Harriet Staples and her sister Louisa were cared for by their aunt Lady Louisa Conolly after their mother, who had "missed a generation for sense," died. Harriet was, "such a merry looking thing" and "a picture of good humour," while Louisa was "as disagreeable a child as ever was." The girls were "eat up with worms" as a result of an unbalanced diet of jelly sugar and butter which was quickly changed

by Lady Louisa.(8)   The "sweet" little Harriet married
the Earl of Clancarty and the disagreeable Louisa wed
Edward Pakenham who, on succeeding to Castletown
through his marriage, changed his name to Conolly.
These were the Conollys living at Castletown when
Arthur arrived at Celbridge to live, not in the great
house, but in the cramped quarters of his tutor, the
Reverend Samuel Greer, in the last house but one on
the left at the approach to Castletown.

Greer was a noted classics scholar whose job it was
to place Arthur's education on a more formal basis and
Celbridge's proximity to Dublin gave easier access to Sir
Philip Crampton, a specialist in the fitting of artificial
limbs who had been introduced to Lady Harriet by Boxwell.
Anne Flemming, Arthur's nurse from infancy, went with
him to Celbridge and in the afternoons, escaping from
Samuel Greer's strict scholastic regime, Arthur used to
ride up to Castletown on his pony led by a "careful lad"
and followed by Anne.   On one such occasion he met
his cousin Mary Conolly for the first time.

"We first became acquainted with Arthur," Mary writes,
"when he was put under the charge of a clergyman
with very high scholastic attainments, the Reverend
Samuel Greer of Celbridge, the village at the gate of
Castletown, my father's place. As well as I can recollect
it must have been about 1839 or 1840 when, on our
return from Donegal, where we usually spent the Autumn
months, as my father was MP for that County, we met
Arthur as we were walking with our nurse in the grounds
of Castletown.   I remember well this first meeting with
the merry looking, fair haired boy riding his pony in
the most fearless way, trying to get it through a very
narrow gate.   Of course he succeeded, as he usually
did in whatever he attempted at that very early age,
to the admiration of us his cousins; and from that day
we became dear friends drawn to him by his singularly
engaging manner, so genial, so manly, so full of sympathy,
a most delightful boy who came into the routine of our
young lives like a sunbeam.   So bright and full of fun
was he that the days when we did not meet him on our

walks were comparatively dull."(9)

Arthur conducted their games from his basket chair on
the back of his pony. "We were all so devoted to him
as to be his most willing subjects. As though he were
a king we would follow his will as law and he often
led us into the most ridiculous pranks." He entertained
them by gripping a sixpence between his stumps and
persuaded the son of the rector of Celbridge to let
him pierce his ears, enjoying the submissiveness of the
victim who was older than he was. He traded on his
cousins credulity and exaggerated his own feats. Mary
Conolly repeats without a hint of disbelief how Arthur,
sitting at his bedroom window in Greer's house with a
fishing rod between his stumps, felt a tug on the line.
A duck had taken the bait and had to be hauled up,
killed, plucked, cooked and eaten before the Greers
found out. Mrs Greer, unamused by his activities, was
strict; but Mary writes, "the sternest could not long
be angry with him," and he used his "merry bright
face and winning ways" to charm the Greer's just as
his grandmother had charmed Lady Louisa Conolly.
"Undaunted courage" and "spirited pluck" made him the
Conolly's hero; and when they left for a prolonged stay
in Paris in 1841 they found the parting "grievous."(10)

Arthur's merriment masked the feelings of a ten year
old boy missing his mother, his brothers and sisters,
particularly Hoddy, and the familiar surroundings of his
home. He felt neglected and excluded. Sadly he wrote
to his mother while she was in Italy, "I suppose you did
did not intend to bring us to Borris this summer therefore
I will see neither Hoddy nor Charley for this reason. I
am very sorry. I suppose you intend going abroad with
Tommy and Charley. May we soon go to Torquay? You
cannot think how happy it would make me to live at
dear Borris again not writing to one another but having
a pleasant chat at home." When his mother criticised
him for not writing longer letters, he hit back half
humourously with a reference to "that very philosophical
story of the pot calling the kettle black."(11)

Lady Harriet was at home in Borris in 1841. O'Connel's campaign for the Repeal of the Act of Union and for the abolition of tithes to the Church of Ireland was gathering momentum, and the Protestant Ascendency was under threat. In the election of 1840 her son-in-law Henry Bruen had been returned as MP for Carlow, defeating the O'Connelites. He attributed his success to the support of the Kavanagh's tenants, two hundred of whom had been 'cooped' at Borris to ensure they supported him.

Commentators have seen Lady Harriet's support for the Tories as evidence of her determination to keep the Parliamentary seat warm for one of her young sons. It was an objective pursued, so it was said, with all the driving force of a Lady Macbeth.(12) In reality the driving force, in her absence, was Doyne, her agent who early in 1841 was presented with silver by the local landlords in return for his support of their candidate. The victory celebrations were deferred until November when Lady Harriet, home from Italy and wishing "to renew her acquaintance with the tenantry, assembled her clans," and "threw open the lofty and spacious baronial halls of Borris to give them a truly Irish Welcome."(12) The Evening News described her "mingling with her tenants," like "Queen Elizabeth going to meet her troops at Tilbury."(13) In the afternoon tenants packed the lawns in front of the House. Young men shinned up slippery poles to win a new hat or bonnet, or ran in races to win a shawl or some other garment as a prize for a wife or sweetheart from Lady Harriet. "Even in the feebleness of old age" some ran in sacks. In the afternoon and "under the canopy of heaven," the tenantry, old and young with their wives, sisters daughters, "and offspring to the third generation," were presented in quick succession to Lady Harriet, flanked by her step-daughters Susan and Grace. At 5 pm two hundred sat down to dinner at tables heavy with rounds and ribs of beef, and legs and shoulders of mutton. There was roast and boiled fowl, plum pudding, pies and tarts and an "abundance of port and sherry" and lemonade for the supporters of the "apostle of temperance". Lady Harriet, Grace, Susan and Lady Louisa presided at the tables and in the evening Lady Harriet opened the Ball, dancing with one of the tenants.

Almost as quickly as she came she was gone again, leaving Arthur at Celbridge. Sir Philip Crampton saw him periodically for the preparation of artificial legs, the fitting of which, on to his six inch stumps, wase uncomfortable and sometimes painful. During these visits to Dublin Arthur stayed with his aunt Louisa and helped his cousin Sarah with her sums. They amused themselves harnessing the dog to a small cart which Arthur drove. The continuing absence of his family was more trying than his physical discomfort and he wrote to his mother in rounded copperplate just after his eleventh birthday.

Dublin, April 13th, 1842

"My Dearest Mamma,

"I suppose this will be my last letter to you as I hope soon to have the happiness of seeing you once more at dear Borris. Anne and I have been obliged to stop in Dublin with Reynolds for a week as he could not make my new legs without me. O dear Mamma you can't think how much I long for your return which I hope will be soon please God. I have written to Tommy and Charley last week begging they would not let you stop at Geneva but to come home quick. I have left my friends at Castletown quite well. Bess Pakenham came there on Thursday but I had to come to Dublin without seeing her. Susan and Grace and all at Borris are quite well. Give my love to my dearest Hoddy; tell her I have bought the nice present which I promised her. I expect Mr Doyne here today to see me. Give my love to all at home.
And I still remain your most affectionate son,

Arthur Kavanagh."

The "new legs" were useless because Arthur's stumps were too short and no more attempts were made to

fit him with artificial limbs. Sir Philip Crampton
distracted him from his disappointment by fostering
his interest in wild life and the two of them made
frequent visits to the Dublin Zoo, laying the foundation
of an interest which lasted throughout Arthur's life.
The greatest compensation however, which Arthur had
at this time, was the abandonment of the basket chair
strapped to his pony's back and its replacement by a
saddle designed by Boxwell. Additional straps buckled
around his thigh stumps and extra girths prevented
slipping, and with reins tight between his arm stumps
he became free to ride alone.

4. ADOLESCENCE

When Arthur returned to Borris he was accompanied by
a tutor, the Reverend David Wood, a meticulous and
humourless man who took his duties seriously. Arthur
continued his studies of Greek, Latin and mathematics
and also developed an interest in navigational skills,
charting tides and currents. He studied the various
species of fish in the local river making copious notes
and became a skilful angler. Wood, who at this point
admired his pupil, describes him crouched at the water's
edge holding his rod firmly between his stumps. "Suddenly
there was a swift powerful flick of his stumps and low
and behold up comes a catch."(1) Arthur, says Wood, was
equally at home fishing in the brook at Borris or on the
Westmeath Lakes. In either case Wood initialled the log
to verify the claim as a safeguard against adolescent
exaggeration. Another form of recreation he enjoyed
was sketching and painting, which he did with pencil or
brush 'hooked' between his stumps or between his teeth
and he wrote sharply to his mother, "I wish you would
buy me some pencils and four or five paint brushes of
different sizes."(2)

Back at Borris the absence of his family seemed more
tolerable but he looked eagerly for his "dearest Mamma's
return and wrote teasingly, "I seize upon the first leisure
to reply to your Ladyship's letter and we will have everything ready for the due reception of your worthy and
much respected Ladyship."(3) The repairs to the cupola
over her room in one of the turrets were, he assured
her, complete and repairs to the others were in process.
These small domes, shown in old prints of the house,
have now disappeared.

The year 1844 was dominated by the trial and conviction
of Daniel O'Connel on charges of conspiracy and unlawful
assembly and by the "unprecedentedly parching weather,"
accompanied by frosts, which aroused fears for the health
of the potato crop.(4) Lady Harriet came home, much to

Arthur's pleasure, and received an ornate card announcing
"Master Arthur Kavanagh and Miss Harriet Kavanagh
and Mrs White will have the honour of waiting on Lady
Harriet Kavanagh at dinner on Sunday at half past four
o'clock. NB We shall expect an excellent dinner".(5)

In November Lady Harriet gave a far more elaborate
entertainment for the labourers, tradesmen and tenants
on the Kavanagh Estates. The large barn at the rear
of the house was "elegantly decorated" with evergreen,
and illuminated by chandeliers and at 5 pm two hundred
and fifty persons sat down to a substantial meal consist-
ing of beef, mutton, ham and fowl. "Many sprightly airs
were performed in excellent style by the musicians."(6)
Proposals of the Health of Lady Harriet and the family
drew cheers and, in the absence of his brothers, Arthur,
aged thirteen, thanked the tenants for the warmth of
their reception of his mother and himself. He proposed
the health of the tenantry, the tables were removed and
there was dancing through to the next morning, with
occasional pauses for refreshment.

Encouraged by his mother, Arthur, took an interest in
the work and development of the estate. He farmed his
own portion, keeping a careful account of his steward-
ship. He sold his wheat for £8 5s 3d and bought two
pigs; his potatoes he sold to Doyne, for £16 0s 0d.
He bought four calves and asked plaintively in a letter
to his mother if the profit had to be given to the poor.

In February 1845 a farming Society was formed on
the Kavanagh estates. Once again five hundred of the
tenantry from Carlow, Wexford and Kilkenny sat down,
a hundred at a time, to the usual "immense rounds
of beef," roast or boiled hams, legs of mutton, bread
and tea. Arthur, Boxwell, Kelly the steward, Morton,
Charley's tutor, and Doyne each presided at one of the
long tables. Arthur watched the "animated scene," and
in the absence, once again of the family, "expressed
satisfaction . . . on being afforded so favourable an
opportunity of interchanging these kindly and mutual
feelings of respect and attachment which ever subsisted

between owner and occupier of the soil."(7) If the
generosity was typical of the Kavanaghs for generations
as local commentators said, the organisation and industry
was typical of the le Poer Trenches.

Doyne spoke from a platform, telling the tenants they
met "by the desire" of Lady Harriet and Thomas their
new landlord "to carry out a design long in contemplation"
- the formation of an Agricultural Society. Lady Harriet,
Doyne said, "was desirous to assist in every useful project
to promote the comfort, happiness and prosperity of the
tenantry;" their young landlord had inherited the virtue
of his ancestors and their attachment to the soil.(8)
He made proposals for drainage and reclamation which
would benefit the tenants but also the landlord. He
urged them to abandon "the trammels of old customs, old
methods and old prejudices," and to adopt more rational
methods of cultivation. He himself had reclaimed fifty
acres in Wexford and was growing turnips to compete
with any in the County. Thomas was offering new
sets of drainage implements and free turnip seed to
all who would drain two acres in two years. The day
concluded with Boxwell offering the apologies of the
parish priest "absent on other business," with cheers for
the landlord and the House of Kavanagh. Two hundred
tenants collected their drainage implements and Doyne
handed over to the new Society £20 from Thomas, and
£5 from Lady Harriet and Arthur.

During July 1845 Doyne had to answer allegations of
neglect, oppression and ejectment, on the Kavanagh
Estates. It was alleged by a Mr Sweetman, "a person
without a local habitation or name," who had married
a local woman and, having failed to ingratiate himself
with the Conservatives, was now filled with zeal to
redress "all the imaginary grievances of his immediate
locality," that eviction was being used as an act of
vengeance against those who had voted against the
landlords' candidate in recent elections. Answering
the allegations, before the Land Commission, Doyne
acknowledged that there had been acts of oppression
notably by a Kavanagh tenant named Corcoran against

those to whom he sub-let and that ejectment notices
had been served. He denied any involvement by the
'head landlord' and laid the difficulties at the door of
the "middlemen." He told the Commission that in his
twenty five years as agent, there had been few changes
in tenancy on the Kavanagh estates. It had been
necessary to evict the "pauper population," as through
sub-letting, "the land swarmed with an idle disorganised
pauper tenantry." Even then, said Doyne, they had
been given the option of leaving peacefully with their
"growing crop," and with compensation. It was false to
say they received no consideration, for all were offered
free passage to America. The industrious were retained
irrespective of religion, and thirty Catholic families had
been placed in "fine slate houses." Of nearly six hundred
tenants on the Estates only twenty were Protestants.
He pointed to the clearing and draining of land and the
replacement of thatch with slate, the landlord providing
free timber, and he believed this was evidence that the
Estate was "one of the most inspiring," in the County.(9)

The terms of tenancy in Ireland differed from those
in England. There was no tenant right, particularly in
the South and most tenancies were on a yearly basis.
Tenants were liable to six months notice. When they
improved their holding its value was raised and the
landlord raised the rent. Some tenants objected to the
landlord carrying out improvements on the grounds that
it too would lead to a rise in rent. It was a system of
disincentive and absolute power wielded justly by some
landlords and unjustly by others and often abused in
their absence by agents and middlemen. "The monstrous
land system in Ireland," wrote Lord Charles Beresford,
"naturally causes the tenants to feel distrust and enmity
towards the landlords;" for though not many landlords
abused their powers, the knowledge that they could
abuse them was alone sufficient to create suspicion and
hostility.(10)

Lady Harriet and Tom contented themselves with the
expression of pious hopes for the well-being of the
tenantry, usually from afar, having confidence in

Doyne's ability to combine protection of the landlords'
interests with appropriate concern for the poor. Arthur
was more involved, even at fourteen, in the working
of the Estate than either of his brothers, and the press
noted that involvement. In the local show he entered a
two year old Bull "which for high breeding and symmetry
could not be excelled," while Delaney, the gardener,
entered turnips "twenty inches long and eighteen inches
in circumference."(11) Arthur enjoyed representing the
family and in the Autumn of 1845 wrote telling them
how well he was doing.

The Harvest Entertainment saw the usual "irrepressible
cheerfulness," and "joyous festivity." Lady Harriet
expressed from some distant part of Europe her concern
to avert the evil of the potato crop failure, and the
"amiable" Tom sent a message looking forward to
being amongst them "to experience their kindness," and
remitted a year's rent on every field they re-claimed.
Their "friend and brother farmer," Arthur Kavanagh
spoke to the four hundred and fifty tenants. He was
happy that the potato crop failure was less severe in
the district than elsewhere but urged them not to be
complacent. He had been experimenting with Morton
and Mrs Doyne on making bread from the sound part
of diseased potatoes. With grated potato, wheaten flour
and soda, bread was being made on the Estate, and "the
proof of the pudding was in the eating," when a large
quantity, "sweet and wholesome," made from four stone
of potatoes was produced.(12) There were cheers for the
bread, and Arthur's health was drunk to more cheering.
The proceedings concluded after Arthur had distributed
"free graters for bread making, which Doyne begged
them to use." Arthur, involved, concerned, admired,
was laying the foundations of a relationship with the
tenants that eluded his mother and brothers. He was
just fourteen.

In October 1845 he was confirmed in the chapel at Borris.
He sat, not in the family pew which at that time was a
gallery entered from the House, but on a low window-
ledge until he was carried to the bishop for the "laying

on of hands." The invocation of the Holy Spirit moved him to introspection and he revealed the first stirrings of the darker side of his nature. He copied the prayer "Almighty God, to whom all hearts are open, all desires known, and from whom no secrets are hid, cleanse the thoughts of our heart by the inspiration of Thy Holy Spirit, that we may perfectly love Thee and worthily magnify Thee." In self examination he accused himself of arrogance, inconsistency, and desiring things he could not have. What things, we are left to conjecture. The confident cheerful youth when alone found "life's way" rough and could identify with the words "though dark my path and sad my lot let me be still and murmur not."(13)

Lady de Vesci leaves us a picture of him on their first meeting. "His head and shoulders reminded me of Bismark's. He took me a walk round the demesne, I on foot, he on a fidgety little mare and seated in a chair saddle. It was hot July weather, and he kept the flies away with unerring aim with his whip, and would not let me open the gate but managed to do all this himself. I never thought of his infirmities . . . his charming voice, his unselfish and remarkable personality led one quite away from them."(14)

Mary McCarthy described him as young and fair-haired with a broad intellectual brow and handsome, with a humorous smile playing about his lips. Only in his deep blue eyes was there any hint of sadness, the merest suggestion of wistful longing. He was strong, lithe, manly, attractive in a frieze-kilt and shooting-jacket, making strong simple nervous shoulders do all the work that ordinary arms could do.

He could ride as straight as any member of the Carlow or Kilkenny hunts, strapped to his saddle with the reins around his stumps and a whip beneath his armpit. As Boxwell foretold there were accidents. While riding in the deer park, his horse bolted and careered three times around the park. According to Arthur, he was just able to guide him when his strength began to fail. He turned the horse towards the demesne wall to stop his "mad

career."(15) The girth gave way and the saddle slipped
and he remembered nothing more until found by one of
his brothers. Whatever happened did not deter him
from riding and he enjoyed telling the story to his
nieces.

Early in 1846 Lady Harriet decided that Arthur's
success in study and sport and on the estate were
not enough. "Arthur is so full of energy and life that
he will only wither away if he stays indefinitely at
Borris. The sole answer for him is to travel as far
afield as possible and to continue his education while
doing so, not merely by diligent study but by special
opportunities of observations and reflections which
foreign travel will give him."(1) She took Arthur to
Paris then on to Florence for a taste of Italian living
and then for an "intensely happy stay" in the Villa
Strozzi in Rome. The experiment was a success and
she decided on a prolonged tour of the Middle East for
the whole family except Charles, who wasn't interested
in travel and who, preparing to join the army, remained
at Borris.

The weather in 1846 was wetter than usual. In early
June there was a heat wave and the combination favoured
the spread of the potato blight for a second year. The
poorer Irish peasants lived off small plots of land, the
rent of which was so inflated that the cereal crops they
grew had to be sold in their entirety to pay the rent.
They hired out their labour, not for a wage but for a
potato crop which was their main food. When that crop
failed they starved. Too weak to work, they could not
pay the rent and many were evicted.

The potatoes around Carlow appeared sound when picked
but gave off an appalling stench when boiled. Typhus
broke out on the Kavanagh Estates in Kilkenny and many
of the population suffered from dysentery. Grain, meal
and butter were carted for exportation along roads lined
by the hungry and Public works were inaugurated to give
the destitute an opportunity to earn enough to feed themselves. According to local tradition the wall surrounding
the demesne at Borris at this time was rebuilt by some
labourers in return for a ration of a meal a day and
conformity to the Protestant religion.

In September 1846 Borris House was alive with preparations for the family's departure for the Middle East. "Shady hats" for Lady Harriet and Hoddy and "shortish skirts," old shooting jackets, guns, the Bible, senna, licorice, pommade divine, David Wood's clerical riding breeches and surprisingly, a copy of Byron's poems for Arthur.(2)

They left Dover on the first of October, crossed to Boulogne, where they stayed at the Hotel de Londres, and left for Paris on the following day. The journey across the plains of Northern France was a cold and misty one. Tom rode on the top of the diligence, Arthur inside with his mother and a group of Americans, who Lady harriet found "clean" and "intelligent."(3)   After resting at the hotel Wagram they left Paris for Chalons where, on the 8th October, they took the steamer to Avignon. The boat was "dirty and comfortless," and crowded with troops on their way to Algeria, and the one hundred and thirty miles took thirteen hours.(3) The rains of Ireland and the mists of the North gave way to the Autumnal warmth of Provence. In Avignon they visited the former Palace of the exiled Popes now serving as a barracks, and sailed from Marseilles on the 14th October. The sea was rough and the passengers sick. On the 16th they were off Sicily and on the 24th they sailed into Alexandria, city of a thousand palaces and the entrance to an exotic new world.

Lady Harriet's plan was to cruise up the Nile as far as the third cataract and then return to Cairo to join a caravan, following in the steps of the Israelites across the Red Sea, and through the desert into the Promised Land.

Cairo was a vibrant city under cover of the hills and ringed by high walls. The skyline was dominated by the citadel and the domes and minarets of the mosques. They were called to prayer as they woke and then joined the merchants and beggars pushing their way past the shops of the gold and silver smiths, the leather workers and silk spinners. In the slave market they were intrigued by the black boys and girls running about, chattering, apparently happily, and kissing their hands and asking them to buy them.

Lady Harriet fussed over the price of chickens at three pence each and mutton at two pence per pound. She hired boats, one for herself and Hoddy and one for Tom, Arthur and Wood, had them submerged to rid them of rats and smaller vermin, and then painted sky-blue. When Wood injured a leg and was unable to accompany the boys on their city jaunts, she felt they were safer in Cairo than in European cities. The Arabs liked Arthur, "they carry him about and help him;"(4) he in turn began to learn their language, meticulously listing words, and acted as the party's faltering interpreter.

Despite an evangelical outlook Lady Harriet was not deterred from satisfying her curiosity about the notorious Cairo dancing girls, drunk on brandy and dancing in half open shirts of transparent gauze. Women as well as men took a delight in their performances which included the sex act in dance. Lady Harriet accompanied the Greek Consul's wife to a performance and wrote to her sister saying, "a notoriously bad woman came jumping into the room and in a most familiar manner embraced the chief ladies and began romping with the young slaves and like the jesters of old, she seemed privileged to make all sorts of impertinent remarks and many broad and evidently not always delicate jokes."(5)

Once embarked on the journey up river Arthur spent the mornings in study with Wood while Lady Harriet read the Old Testament. In the afternoons Tom and Arthur fished from the bank or the boat while Hoddy collected flowers. Tom shot pigeons perched on the roof-tops of the houses of the villages they passed. Arthur longed to be allowed to shoot but was forbidden. They savoured the softness and lushness of an Egypt little changed since the days of the Pharoes. They watched the white egrets feeding and the heron and stork standing motionless in the swamps, and were intrigued by the temples and mud-brick villages inhabited by peasant farmers with a lifestyle unchanged for five thousand years. To all of them it was magic.

In mid-January they moored their house-boats between Luxor and Karnak, already popular as an English watering place. Lady Harriet and the others went ashore leaving Arthur resting in the sun on his own boat with his back against the gunwale of another. A sudden heaving of the waters separated the two craft and Arthur fell into the river. He was pulled out by onlookers, and though half-drowned, he survived undaunted. As Boxwell had wished, fear was alien to his nature. Lady Harriet found the whole trip had "quite enough danger to make it an exciting business."(6)

While Lady Harriet and her children wintered on the Nile, Ireland suffered from heavy snow falls and fierce gales; roads were impassable and horses sank in drifts; starving orphans were turned away from the work houses and starving dogs tore the bodies of their masters to pieces. "Never in my life," wrote Commander Caffyn of the sloop 'Scourge', "have I seen such wholesale misery."(7) When the new session of Parliament opened on the 19th January 1847 the Queen seemed downcast and sorrowful, her voice trembled and fell low as she spoke of the sufferings of the Celtic population and commended the patience and exemplary resignation with which they bore their hardship.

Back in Cairo Lady Harriet's group joined three other parties in a caravan of sixty camels crossing into Sinai at one of the points associated with the flight of the Israelites from Egypt. Riding on camels, they turned southwards, as did Moses and his people, avoiding the shortest route parallel to the Mediterranean coast. They followed an ancient beaten track made by slave gangs who had been digging for copper and turquoise in the Sinai mountains since 3000 BC. They passed through barren scrub land to Elim where "there were twelve wells of water and three score and ten palm trees."(8) It was here that quails came up and covered the camp and where lay the mysterious dew. "When the dew was gone, behold upon the face of the wilderness there lay a small round thing, as small as the hoar frost on the ground."(9) This was the manna which the Israelites ate at Moses' command and which, along with the quails, are still an unexceptional occurrence; manna, as sweet as honey, being a secretion of the Tamansk tree which crystalises when pierced by a plant-louse.

From Elim they went into the Wilderness of Sin, a mountainous expanse of torrid plateau, several hundred metres above the Red Sea. Not a breath of wind nor a breeze cooled the travellers' brows and only the camel thorns broke through the yellow sand.

It was a hard but magnificent journey. They rose at 4 am, travelling in the cool of the morning, sheltered in the mid-day heat and dined at 6 pm. The Sinai massif rose before them from the plateau. "Precipitous cliffs of pink and mauve granite thrust their way upwards to the blue sky. Between them sparkle slopes and gorges of pale amber and fiery red, streaked with lead coloured veins of porphery and dark green bands of felspar."(10) Leaving the 'Mount of Moses' they turned North along the West shore of the Gulf of Akabar, and in Akabar itself negotiated for protection from brigands before venturing on to Petra. It was a place with an evil reputation visited only by the most intrepid travellers at this time, and in the Spring of 1847 the pitiless heat was replaced by flood waters which rushed down the gullies causing the travellers to wade ankle deep in mud.

Lady Harriet noted that Arthur had become very fond of the bedouin whom she considered good natured and hospitable "though they are ferocious and will attack travellers."(11) She found them to be chivalrous and attributed the party's safety to the presence of women; one of the sheiks offered to build her a fort if she would remain with him as his wife. The bedouin were in turn, intrigued by the fair-haired boy who, without arms or legs could ride, and who could also speak their language.

After thirty six days the travellers were still rising
at 4 am, breakfasting, packing and loading, and moving
on by 5.30. One day, during an afternoon rest, Lady
Harriet gave a tea party for the bedouin, at the end of
which they all stood while she led the singing of 'God
Save the Queen'. In the early evenings they pitched
their tents and made their beds; the camp was a very
busy place until after dinner when Arthur and the men
sat around the fire smoking before retiring to sleep.

At Hebron, like Moses' scouts, they saw the Promised
Land. To the west was Jerusalem, to the north Samaria,
Galilee and the snow clad peaks of Hermon. Arthur
was appreciative of the change from "the arid sands
of Africa, to the grassy plains, wooded mountains and
silver streams of the Land of Promise." "It seems as
if it were a dream, a fairy land!" He wrote to his
brother Charles, "Picture to yourself gardens of apricots
and pomegranates, vineyards and olive yards, intersected
with sparkling brooks and silver fountains, where the
rose and the myrtle in full bloom send their fragrant
scents to the cloudless heaven and perfume the balmy
air with their delicious odours."(12) He was sure
Charles would enjoy the East "immensely" - with "the
most delicious fruit and everything enjoyable."

It was not just the fruit that attracted him to the
Land of Promise.

> "Where the citrus and olive are fairest of fruit,
> And the voice of the nightingale never is mute,
> Where virgins are soft as the roses they twine,
> And all, save the spirit of man is divine."

"It would charm you to see their beautiful eyes . . . "
he wrote,

> "These eyes dark charm 'twere vain to tell!
> But gaze on these of the gazelle,
> It will assist my fancy well . . . "(13)

The signs of Arthur's stirring sensuality did not escape
either of his brothers and Charles wrote to Tom saying

that he suspected Arthur, "who seems to have fallen
in love with Arab beauties," was "fishing in very deep
waters indeed."(14)

At Hebron they changed camels for horses and Arthur
bought a mount named Dougal M'tavish from the Governor.
Dougal was "a nice little fellow," well behaved though
he fought "with another in the party of the same sex."(15)

In Jerusalem at Easter, Arthur was present at the
annual dispute between Christians of the Latin and Greek
rites over who removed the alter cloth in the Calvary
Chapel at the beginning of the Latin Liturgy. He wrote
approvingly of the intervention of the Turks:

"At that moment the Pasha himself, with a reinforcement of troops marched into the chapel and up to the
altar. He addressed both parties on the propriety of
peace at such a time and exhorted the Greeks to allow
the Latin function to proceed in a proper manner.
But, being angrily answered by both parties, he said he
would march off to prison any person who broke the
peace and that as he was desirous that no cause of
discord should remain, he would himself remove the
altar cloth, which he did immediately with the
greatest coolness and dignity".(16)

Travelling northwards still sleeping in tents, they saw
that shepherds, even now, watched their flocks by night
around Bethlehem, and that fishermen cast their nets
into the waters of Galilee as in the time of Christ. At
the end of May Lady Harriet marked time in Beyrouth,
wondering whether to return to Ireland or spend another
year in the Middle East. "We do not know," Arthur wrote
to his brother Charles, "whether we are to leave for
Constantinople and spend another year in our wanderings
or else go direct home. The next letters will decide
us We have had a jolly time of it."(17) The boys took
stock of their acquisitions. Tom had a Turkish costume,
"all embroidered with gold," and a white silk prayer mat
belonging to Mehemet Ali Pasha; Arthur had a Bedouin
costume. In addition they had Arab guns, one "nearly

six feet in the barrel, all in-laid with silver," sabres, scimitars, knives, shields of giraffe and crocodile skin, spears and Nubian daggers; everything to delight their imagination.

News from Ireland was bad. In the West, Bartholomew Kavanagh, a young curate in Westport and a distant kinsmen of the Kavanaghs of Borris, being descended from the transplanted Murtagh of Castletown, was anointing forty dying parishioners daily. The fever epidemic was at its most virulent and the work-houses overcrowded; the sick lay naked on straw beside the dead. There was no fire to warm them, no medicine to heal them, and no one to bring them food or water.

Lady Harriet decided not to return to Ireland but to travel on to Constantinople, where amusement and surprise were mingled when she visited the wife of the Pasha. She wrote telling her sister, "The first arrangement she made was that we were all to sleep together. I must have looked surprised for she said, 'mais surement vous ne craignez pas de dormir avec une femme Turk?'"(18) Having visited the Black Sea shores as far as Trezibond and being quarantined at Smyrna, where their money was only accepted after it had been passed through vinegar on tongues, they arrived back in Beyrouth on the 24th September to learn that the health of Lady Harriet's mother, the Dowager Lady Clancarty, was failing. Lady Harriet wrote hoping that her mother would see the Will of God in her sufferings, and gain a sense "of His mercy and love."(19)

They planned now to return to Cairo by the short route and spend a second winter on the Nile. "We have bought our horses for the journey to Cairo - six," Arthur wrote, "I have a very nice horse indeed. I gave seventeen hundred piastras for him. He has a true Arab mark on his ear, and everybody I have shown him to says that if not entirely, he is very nearly pure Arab breed. He stands about fifteen hands, has a beautiful head and a fine ear, long nose, almost a milk white coat shining like glass; his limbs are fine without a puff; his eye and the expression of his countenance fiery, yet sweet - an odd phrase to use about a horse, but I do not know any other which expresses what I want so well. He is the admiration of everybody here. Mamma even thinks he will be worth taking home." When Arthur came out of his tent each morning the "fiery steed" would lick his face, and he used to sit under him for shade at "luncheon time" and feed him bread, which he took gently, "without hurting me."(20)

In Jerusalem for the second time Lady Harriet had an attack of the ague, the only note of sickness on the whole tour, and paused by the Pool of Siloam, where Jesus sent the blind man to wash, after having cured him. In an olive grove near Bethlehem they roasted a whole sheep for dinner, unaware that at Buckingham Palace Queen Victoria was rationing the bread in deference to her starving Irish subjects.

In Cairo, in early December, news of continuing famine in Ireland provoked Lady Harriet to write to her brother and sister-in-law. "Why famine exists at all I cannot understand. The harvest was good and I hear stories that foreign corn supplies are overflowing. I can only put it down to bad government."(21) It was a simplistic but common view failing to understand the enfeebled peasants' inability to earn enough to buy corn and the government's decision to cut off aid and allow "market forces" to regulate matters.

Neither news of the famine, nor of her mother's death, deterred Lady Harriet from following her plans to spend another winter on the Nile, which she described as "very healthful."(22) While waiting she enjoyed the junketing in Cairo. She wrote to her sister Louisa describing how she went in procession "through the dark streets of the city led by a black boy in a blue suit and white turban carrying a long pole topped by a cage filled with burning sticks. He ran as fast as he could, with all the ladies and gentlemen on donkeys going at full gallop with the donkey boys running behind."(23) She again hired two boats, one for herself and Hoddy on which they dined, usually in the open air, and received guests, and the other for Tom, Arthur and Wood. She sent her sister a small plan of their "little home on the Nile," telling her that when, on warm evenings they walked on the river bank, they imagined their family back in Ireland "in a closed room with a good fire trying to keep warm."(24)

Arthur was delighted when, on this second Nile trip, he was allowed to shoot. He had practised without hooks or gadgets by throwing his gun, without trigger guard, across his left stump, which supported the stock, and flicking the trigger with his right stump. It was a procedure that required great patience. Lord Morton, who had now joined the party, refused Arthur's requests to be allowed to shoot until he had almost killed himself with a sawn-off shot gun surreptitiously borrowed. Tom, usually loyal to his younger brother, argued that if he could land a trout he could handle a gun, admitting however, that in fishing the fish is the target whereas in shooting the target is the world. Lord Morton was given the job of persuading Lady Harriet to permit Arthur to shoot, and Tom hardly helped by assuring her that after Arthur had shot his third bedouin they would abandon the experiment. Tom later wrote of Arthur, " . . . he has shot a great many wild geese and snipe. He shoots much better than Mr Wood who began about the same time as he did and can hit a flying bird quite well. His shooting is quite as wonderful as his riding."(25) Arthur shot from the boat and sometimes from a donkey on the bank and became so absorbed in the sport that Lady Harriet and Hoddy had to apologise to their cousins for his failure to reply to letters. "He would rather shoot pigeons than answer letters."(26)

On March 2nd they arrived back in Cairo. In the souks Arthur was reunited with some of his bedouin friends. The hirsute tribesmen ran up to him, threw their arms around him and kissed him, as charmed by him as the Conolly children had been much earlier. Arthur was overjoyed that Hadji Mohammed and their two Syrian gazelles, "one black and one deeply stained with henna," were going home to Borris with him, but he parted in tears from his "fiery steed" which had carried him from Beyrouth.

On April 10th they arrived in Marseilles having decided to avoid Italy because of the political uncertainties. The monarchy of Louis Philip had perished in Paris; there had been bloodshed in Berlin, and demonstrations in Vienna had led to Metternick's fall. In London seven thousand troops guarded public buildings and the court had moved to Osborne. The Prince Consort considered Ireland still to be dangerous and Lady Harriet hesitated about returning, considering instead, a visit to Spain. She and Hoddy were keen to go there, while Arthur and Tom hankered after North Africa as a sportsman's paradise. Waiting in Marseilles Arthur noted "thousands" of troops passing his window and complained that he heard nothing but the 'Marseilles Hymn'. "A great panic has struck all commercial men," he wrote, "the bankers refuse to cash any bills whatever. The shops are all shut at sunset, because there is no demand for their articles, they do not care to burn their lights for nothing. All public works have been stopped because the Government have no money to pay the workmen. There is a general dissatisfaction on account of the election being put off. So much for the good of a revolution."(27)

Despite the problems, they decided to return to Ireland. On April 20th the Court Circular announced with some inaccuracy "Lady Harriet Kavanagh and Thomas Kavanagh Esquire are expected early in the ensuing month after a tour through Egypt, India, Turkey, Greece etc. Mr Kavanagh will attain his majority next August when he intends to reside permanently on his Estates. The event will be marked with joy by his numerous tenantry."(28)

Even while absent, Lady Harriet had swept the board at the Athy Horticultural show, thanks to her faithful gardener, Delaney. She gained first prize for the greatest variety of ceneraria, for the most tastefully arranged cut-flowers, for the best specimens of green-house plants, the rarest fuchsias, and potatoes "large and free from taint or spot."(29) Her cucumbers, and asparagus were superior to all others, her eating and cooking apples gained second prize but she was unplaced in the rhubarb.

The Kavanaghs landed at Kingstown, from Liverpool, in mid-May. They had been absent for eighteen months. On the day of their return, Borris "presented a most animated appearance from an early hour."(30) The temperance bandsmen piled their instruments into a brake pulled by four horses, and drove half way to Bagenalstown, where they took up position by the road side, amongst the waiting crowds. As Lady Harriet's carriage was sighted they struck up 'Home Sweet Home'. Lady Harriet and Tom were "gratified" by the welcome and the bandsmen led the procession along the straight and undulating road into Borris. As the carriages turned into the gateway of the House, the band, not entirely appropriately, played "God Save the Queen". If any rushed to slam their doors on this occasion, they did so unnoticed.

That evening the houses of the more affluent citizens, Dr Boxwell, Father Doyle, and Captain Sweeny, were illuminated, and Delaney's house was decked with "exotic flowers." The Carlow Sentinel, with little justification, spoke of Tom as a young gentleman who had "manifested a more than ordinary attachment to his native land."(31)

6. WILD OATS

By the spring of 1848 the capitulation of European governments faced by violence had led the Young Irelanders to believe that no government could any longer resist a mob. They had been organised in 1842 as a political and secular movement to unite Irish patriots irrespective of creed or class. They sought to free peasants from their landlords and Ireland from English rule. They wanted fair rents, security of tenure and free sale of tenants' rights. In May of 1848 their leader, John Mitchell, an advocate of revolution, was tried and sentenced to transportation. His place was taken by the young Protestant Old-Harrovian, William Smith O'Brien, who had sat in Parliament at Westminster for fourteen years and had concluded that Westminster would never legislate in Ireland's interest.

Amidst whispers of rebellion Arthur and his family began resettling at Borris. He spent much of his time reminiscing about his Middle Eastern tour at Oak Park, the home of his half-sister and her husband Colonel Bruen, where he had fun with his nieces and their ponies, driving a four in hand with one of the girls beside him, pelting the leading horse with small stones to make it go faster.

In July he went to stay with his great aunt, the Dowager Lady Ormonde at Garryricken. Here he began riding out alone at night, ostensibly scouring the countryside for rebels, just as his great uncle the Archbishop of Tuam had done. Rebels were active in the area and Arthur claimed to have discovered one of their camps and to have been pursued by their 'cavalry'. Only the speed and cross country prowess of his good horse Bunny saved him from capture, their horses being unable to take the fences to which he fearlessly put his own. "He rode," it was said, "on a full moonlit night over the stone walls, down the mountain side making the stones fly at every stride, across the brook and through the swamps till he had fairly baffled all pursuit and could sit still and laugh at his ease."(1) It was a good story that undoubtedly enlivened the evening for his nieces but the rebels were armed with pikes, scythes and old guns and had few horses of any worth.

Father Fitzgerald the parish priest of Ballingary took another view of his outings. The "rising," which was merely the siege of the widow Cornmac's cottage with shots exchanged between the O'Brienite rebels and the police, was in his parish and he was well informed on the activities of the local people. He accepted that Arthur did ride out alone at night, not as a government spy, "but on many occasions merely to engage in mid-night meetings with a certain young woman who had taken a fancy to the hapless crippled youth. I do not suppose for one moment that his family had any idea that the moon had conjured up for him other and more romantic attractions than that of finding a few of O'Brien's followers."(2) If rumours of these activities at Garryricken reached Lady Harriet and the Reverend David Wood, they chose at this point to ignore them.

The further failure of the potato crop meant another year without rent for the landlords. Evicted tenants in the West of Ireland lived in banks and in ditches until starvation drove them into the work-house. Mr Michael Shaughnessey, the Assistant Barrister, a judicial officer appointed by the Crown, was frequently asked for sentences of transportation by young men convicted of theft so that they might escape starvation. "I am satisfied," he said, "that they had no alternative but starvation or the commission of crime." Some months had now gone by since feeding the children had been stopped, and naked little creatures with hair standing on end, eyes sunken and bones protruding through their skin, roamed the streets.(3)

Tom Kavanagh came of age on the 10th of August 1848, when six hundred tenants gathered to celebrate in an "encampment" on the lawns in front of Borris House. He presided at a table 62 feet in length from which others radiated and all of which were covered with awnings of strained canvas decorated with Delaney's exotic flowers. In front of him was the Charter Horn, symbol of the Kavanagh's authority. It was an ivory drinking horn, tipped with brass, which had been given to Donnell son of Dermot MacMurrough in 1175 when he submitted to the English crown. The iron Crown of Leinster and the Horn had been taken to Trinity College Dublin for safe keeping at the time of the rising of 1798. The crown had been lost but the horn had been returned to Borris. The guests at the celebration ate a variety of meats and fowl and drank ale and cider drawn from casks placed at the end of each table. The press noted the presence among the servants, of "an Arab in full costume, a fine intelligent man."(4) It was Arthur's favourite Hadji Mohammed, who had returned with them from the Middle East.

In the evening Tom opened the Ball for the tenantry by dancing with his mother. Lord and Lady Clancarty, Lord and Lady Ormonde and Lord Dunlo were among the guests and Charles, now in the 3rd Buffs, was present with his brother officers. At dusk, bonfires burned on Mount Leinster and the House was thrown open to all comers. Eight thousand people crowded the village streets. From the drawing room the ladies watched the fireworks and among them was Miss Fanny Irvine with whom Arthur had fallen in love. Whether she was the only lover is uncertain but by the Spring of 1849 Arthur was again "fishing in dangerous waters." The Reverend David Wood was alarmed enough to initiate "a long and serious talk" with Lady Harriet about Arthur's activities.

"The rumours of last summer seem most unfortunately to have reached Borris again. Any suggestion that Arthur is pursuing undesirable friendships with unsuitable females cannot fail to make both him and the family look ridiculous. It remains to be seen whether a lecture or a prolonged period of travel overseas may be the maximum required to restore a sense of proportion. My responsibility is to convince myself whether he is merely philandering, which would be reprehensible or

- 48 -

in earnest which would be deplorable."(5) Fanny Irvine
had gone through a form of betrothal or a clandestine
marriage at Newtown Park; and as Arthur subsequently
referred to her in a letter to his sister as "my dearest
wife,"(6) it seems almost certain that he was the man
involved. If Hoddy knew about it then it is likely that
Lady Harriet and Wood also knew.

Arthur was changing. He was prone to outbursts of rage
and his mother found him at best "disrespectful" and at
worst rushing into "a wild vortex of idle pleasures."(7)
She cast herself in the role of a weak woman unsupported
by a husband or father and unable to cope with a recalc-
itrant son. She adopted Wood's suggestion that Arthur
should travel abroad for as long as was necessary to
resolve the problem. She acknowledged to herself, that
she was sending him away and that it caused her pain.
It was decided that Tom who, a year earlier, "manifested
a more than ordinary attachment to his native land,"(8)
and who had come to live among his tenants as did his
ancestors, should accompany his brother. Arthur's friends
regretted his departure and he himself disliked the idea
of banishment, particularly as he had not been told why
he was going.

7. EXILE - RUSSIA

On the fourth of June 1849 Arthur, Tom, David Wood
and William Wright their servant, sailed from Kingstown
in the "Iron Duke." Arthur sketched the ship in the
margin of his diary. It was a Summers day and "a
beautiful passage" and for two of the four men, the
fading hill town, with its churches and houses tumbling
down the slopes to the sea, was their last sight of
Ireland.

They arrived in Liverpool at four thirty in the morning
and booked in at Fountains Hotel in St James' Street
twelve hours later. After a brief visit to Kew and a
concert at the Exeter Hall they sailed for Copenhagen
which they found very dull. Arthur's parting pleasure
was a letter from his old nurse Anne Flemming.

During the crossing the upright Wood became involved
with a Swiss governess. Tom wrote to his mother a
description of the dark-eyed girl gazing into the sea
and feeding the fishes. Wood, he said, soon distracted
her, wrapped her in his cloak and plied her with brandy
and water. The humourless tutor wrote his own defensive
account of the incident to Lady Harriet. "Arthur, whether
in joke or not, I don't know, and Tom also, tell me they
say such-and-such things of me in their letters to you,
which I should be very sorry if you took literally."(1)
"Arthur too," he told Lady Harriet, "used to sit close
to the girl and beg her to play the piano to them, and
now they both declare that I was the attentive one."(2)

Beyond reach of their mother's strictures, Tom and
Arthur were not inclined to be ruled by Wood. During
a brief stay in Norway they were invited to join a Mr
Crowe and his family for dinner; Wood was shocked to
find that even though it was the Sabbath, about twenty
people arrived and began dancing. "I could not resist
the National habit," he wrote, "but contented myself
with a simple expression of my feelings on the subject

by withdrawing to the library to read." Arthur and Tom remained with the dancers, and a peeved Wood noted, "Miss Crowe was in the party, a good natured girl with whom Arthur got on capitally; don't let the young ladies in Ireland be jealous - she is engaged."(3)

While in Sweden they learned that their Russian visas, given in London, were invalid. The British Minister was unhelpful and the Swedes, Arthur thought, were good only at bowing and spitting.

When the party finally arrived in St Petersburg it was "great fun." There were balls, masquerades, and dinner parties; Tom and Arthur wrote to Hoddy asking her to persuade their mother to visit Russia. The days were hot so they drove out in the evening in caravans of sledges, some drawn by horses, some by reindeer, to the Ice Hills where, after moonlit suppers, they took sledges down the slopes.

With an eye for feminine beauty and also a degree of adolescent exaggeration, Arthur recorded that the Grand Duchess Olga was "quite the most beautiful woman in Russia, and one of the handsomest women I have ever seen."(4)

The journey to Moscow was an eventful one; a wheel of their carriage caught fire making Arthur very aware of the eight pounds of gunpowder under his seat; the carriage left the road and sank into a ditch and finally an axle broke. The latter incident was on Tom's birth-day and Arthur treated him to a bottle of Champagne, although it did not escape Tom's notice that while he paid for it, Arthur and Wood drank it.

Arthur found Moscow "more ugly than curious, with streets badly paved and houses decaying from neglect rather than age."(5) The food, however, was "capital." For dinner they had caviar, soup, sirloin of beef, peas, mushrooms, carrots, and potatoes "dosed with squash - a sort of fermented liqueur made from potatoes." There were plums and pineapples, mulled ale, iced champagne, bottles of "capital claret," pipes of "good tobacco," and coffee. "All in all most capital."(6)

While in Moscow they became involved with a French actress, Mademoiselle Dubois. They suspected her and her English associate, a man called Mitchinson, of trying to rob them, and after an evening of drinking they visited her flat to serenade her. Her response was to empty "a very dirty liquid from a very dirty utensil" over them.(7) In revenge they stormed the house. While Arthur kept watch from the carriage, led by a young blood named Lilley, they broke down the door, smashed the staircase and made their get-away just before the police arrived.

In three months they spent five hundred pounds and Wood confided to Lady Harriet that he was afraid to ask Tom to account for it. Tom, now on the defensive, wrote to his mother telling her that Russia was the most expensive country in the world and his troubled conscience indicated that the money would have been better spent among his own people. Arthur, likewise, was troubled about conditions in Ireland, and wrote, "I trust things will continue to improve and if ever I should see its dear old face again I may come to a country no longer the seat of famine, misery and wretchedness but enjoying the blessings which everyone who knows it and loves it well, as I do, would rejoice to see her possessed of." He asked his mother to seek out an old servant, Morgan Brennan, and not let him starve, and to pay two others the extra wages he promised for building his boat.(8)

Arthur's thoughts were on the young women he had left behind, and the Queen's visit to Ireland provided a pretext for enquiring about them. Taking advantage of the improving situation, Queen Victoria sailed for Cork on the 27th July. An anxious Lady Lyttelton watched "England's fate afloat" from the windows of Osborne House as the ship taking the Queen and her family disappeared from view.(9) Despite the privations of the Famine years, when the Queen sailed into Cork "in the golden light of a summer sunset," bonfires blazed in welcome on the hills. On the 4th August she was safely in Vice-regal Lodge and in the reception party was the Kavanaghs' friend and medical advisor Sir Philip Crampton. In Dublin houses were decked with flowers and "the lamp posts black with living clusters," as her Irish subjects struggled to see her. The Royal party drove "not in a gorgeous train of state carriages preceded by music," but in "three beautiful but private carriages." At Trinity College she admired the book of St Moling, in its silver case, and the Charter Horn of the Kavanaghs. Charles' regiment - he was now in the 7th Hussars - escorted her to the Levee held at Dublin Castle, and Charles was presented to the Queen by Lord Clancarty. She wore a "robe of exquisitely shaded Irish poplin of emerald green, richly wrought with shamrocks in gold embroidery."(10)

At the 'Drawing Room' on the following Thursday she wore "pink poplin embroidered with shamrocks."(11) In a letter Arthur enquired if his cousin Frances Forde Leathly was there and then went on to enquire about Fanny Irvine who, he had heard, was in "bad spirits."

Neither Lady Harriet nor Fanny Irvine attended the Queen's 'Drawing Room'. Lady Harriet had "neither curiosity, nor loyalty enough to go to the expense and trouble of being presented to her myself," and she sent Hoddy in her place. It was an odd response from the woman who had led the bedouin in singing 'God save the Queen' in the desert. Hoddy joined the press of 2000 who waited, each with two large cards bearing their names, packed in a stifling waiting room. It was an ordeal for the Queen's guests and the Queen found it "not quite pleasant" for her hand, as her sweating subjects were presented.(12)

Fanny Irvine, who was in disgrace, was forbidden by her mother to attend the Queen's Drawing Room and Lady Harriet attributed her poor looks and bad spirits to this disappointment or to Arthur's absence. Through Hoddy he sent Fanny a message, "give her my love and tell her, my dearest wife, that I have her precious verbena safe and hope to bring it home and exchange it for a more substantial and lasting proof of her unalterable affection."(13)   Hoddy's reply was terse: "I sent your message to Fanny Irvine but am afraid she has none of the same sort to send you. She does not consider the ceremony she went through at Newtown Park in the slightest degree binding."(14)

From Moscow the group travelled to one of the world's largest fairs at Nijni-Novgorod. Here they went nightly to the cafes to watch the gypsies dancing. Arthur liked their singing but was disappointed with their looks, though one or two impressed him with their fiery eyes, dark complexions and hair like jet. "They lead an odd life,"(15) he wrote, after one of the few erasures in his diary, and he joined in their dancing, imitating, as best he could on his short stumps, the Cossack leap. Wood and Tom also joined in, though Wood wrote hastily to Lady Harriet to assure her it was involuntary on his part. The lifestyle of the gypsies, he thought, might be considered indecorous, even barbaric, but in reality they behaved quite well. He did many things, he said, for the sake of the boys, that he would never do at home and in this way he could influence what he could not forbid.

Although they had been away only three months, Tom and Arthur were anxious to return to Borris. Tom pleaded Arthur's cause saying he promised to be sober and steady, but Wood, conscious of his mandate to keep Arthur away for as long as it took to solve the "problem", was intent on travelling to India. Tom challenged Wood to a game of billiards; if he won he would return home; if he lost he would travel to India with Arthur and the others. Tom lost but Wood declined to accept a decision based on the outcome of a game of billiards. In a second game, if Tom lost he vowed he would travel as far as Persia with the others. He did lose and, according to Wood, accepted his lot gracefully, but in a letter to his mother, he felt he had decided his fate in a game of billiards.

At Nijni-Novgorod they made provision for travelling 'light' down the Volga and embarked with six port-manteaux, two cases of sherry, carpet bags, brandy, tea, guns, hat boxes and a book box. The journey to Astrakhan took three tedious weeks. Every evening they "lay to" and sailed again at sunrise; a precaution necessary to avoid the inumerable sand banks in the river. In the daytime they gazed at the endless stretches of sand and water, shot duck, teal, wild geese, widgeon and cormorants and grumbled at the idleness, and stupidity of the Russian sailors. The weather was cold and showery contrasting with the heat of Moscow. Arthur read Shakespeare, encouraged by Wood, to store his memory with something more wholesome than the "sickly sentiment of Byron, whose works they regret to have left behind."(16)

At night they slept on the floor with their cloaks as pillows, having abandoned their air-beds, one of which had precipitated Arthur onto the floor as he struggled to adjust it. The food was poor; no more caviar, only boiled cabbage and beef and potatoes cooked in oil.

On 24th September they arrived at Astrakhan. The frost was so sharp they decided to travel to Persia, not via the Caucasus, but across the Caspian. The boat they took was crowded; Tom and Wood got a cabin, Arthur and William Wright slept on the floor in the mess. It was a stormy journey and most of the crew were sick. Arthur produced a bottle of brandy to raise their morale; the only remaining crewman got drunk and in the morning they were drifting, with little idea of their position.

8.   PERSIA

On the 9th of October 1849 they landed at Gawzaw,
a village on the southern shore of the Caspian Sea.
The journey on horseback to Teheran took them through
jungle said to abound with lions, tigers and wild boar,
but they encountered only pheasants, hare and jackal.
At times the jungle appeared impenetrable. Wild 'rope-
wire' threaded itself into a net around the giant oaks
with "the beautiful acacia growing up in the greatest
luxuriance."(1)

Some times they slept in sheds with bats for company,
other times they slept out in the rain. They rose at
dawn, set off without breakfast and rode all day except
for periodic halts for their Muslim guides to pray. They
were "caged" and pelted with rotten eggs and oranges at
Astrabad and refused entry to the inn because they were
Christians. They were delivered from brigands, Arthur
supposed, because one of the guides began to "tell his
beads vigorously."(2) Some nights they bathed "nearly
dead with hunger,"(3) eating only a portion of chicken
each, "meagre fare for hungry fellows."(4) One evening
they ate sixteen eggs for want of anything better.

With wet clothes drying on their backs and plagued
by mosquitoes, they began the ascent of the Elburz
Mountains. Arthur was moved by the magnificent
scenery and undaunted by the "villainous road" which
was impassable except to local ponies. For thirty five
minutes they edged their way along a narrow ledge.
On one side the rock rose vertically above them, and
on the other fell away some four hundred feet. Arthur's
mount slipped twice and both times he believed he was
about to fall into the chasm. The meticulous Wood
dismounted, took out a tape measure and measured the
path; it was fourteen inches wide.

As they came down on the other side the rain was
continuous; it was cold and misty and there were

disputes with their guides about food. There were some compensations; on 21st October Arthur recorded in his diary, "I shot grouse."

It was a miserable journey and Arthur was low in spirits. Wood chose, at this point, to tell him the reasons for his exile. "It was not until we were on the road between Astrabad and Teheran, my dear mother, that I was told your reason for sending me abroad. One reason I knew - that was the idle good for nothing life I was leading, but disrespect for you never crossed my mind, so blind are we to our faults. I have thought much of it since . . . it did not arise from any feeling of disrespect but my own thoughtlessness and hot temper which I cannot command."(5) He concluded dutifully, saying he was ready to return home or continue his travels according to his mother's wishes.

On arrival in Teheran the party was attacked and pelted with stones and had to be rescued by attachees from the British Embassy. William Wright and then Arthur became ill with fever and it was three weeks before they could travel again. Arthur felt the cold; the temperature was now around 15 degrees and William complained a lot, so irritating Arthur by his "unmanly" behaviour, that he threatened to send him home. "William again pleaded his inability to go on, declaring we should have to bury him by the roadside, so we decided to stop again."(6)

There was a brief respite for them in Sultania where Arthur enjoyed champagne and a good dinner with a European family. From there they rode to Tabriz. At times Arthur was barely able to sit on his horse. On the 18th of November William was found to have frost-bite and it was decided to send him back to Ireland. Although irritated by his servant's lack of stamina, Arthur wrote to Lady Harriet asking her to re-instate him in his old job.

In Tabriz Arthur met Prince Malichus Mirza, whom he judged to be about thirty five, considerably above six feet, with a magnificent beard and jet black eyes.

He was a "perfect gentleman," spoke French fluently
and lived in the European style. Arthur was sure his
mother would like him. Unknown to Arthur, Mirza had
been Richard Burton's mentor when he was collecting
information on Eastern erotica and was associated with
him in preparation of the Khama Sutra. Arthur enjoyed
the Prince's champagne and good cuisine but became
too ill, with bouts of dysentery, to travel further. Tom
and Wood decided to ride to Tiflis in Georgia, leaving
Arthur in Tabriz.

Letters from home had been few since they had embarked
on the Volga. Even then Arthur was pining to go home
and Hoddy was too preoccupied to write to him because
of her courtship with a Colonel Middleton. On Christmas
Day 1849 Arthur wrote, "Between sickness and loneliness
etc I spent the most miserable of Christmas days."(7)
On New Years Day 1850 he felt well enough to get up,
but by the evening was half conscious. Malichus moved
him into his harem to be cared for by an old black
slave, who became devoted to him. Arthur regarded
Malichus as the handsomest man he had ever seen, and
Malichus presented Arthur to the women of the harem
as a "young blonde god."(8) He found the harem well
conducted and the women showed him great kindness.
They were "well mannered" and "civilised" and he felt
something in common with a fair-haired Armenian,
who told him how she longed to be back home with her
family. The only disadvantage was the women's tendency
to squabble over who would nurse him on their knees.

When Tom and Wood returned from Georgia, the latter
with dyed hair, Malichus was holding Arthur incommun-
icado. Wood's enquiries were met with evasiveness; he
concluded from the Prince's "indelicate gestures" that
Arthur was living in the harem. Wood was outraged
at the thought of Arthur "incarcerated" under the
Prince's jurisdiction in a "place of pagan pleasure" and
"unchaperoned amid a score or more of dubious females
who even with allowances for charity's sake can only be
deemed concubines."(9) He tried to enlist the help of
the British Minister with talk of Arthur being kept in

a claustrophobic prison with a mysterious room that was always locked. Wood's belief that the Prince was a corrupting influence seemed to be confirmed when he told him that Arthur would go out into the world much better equipped to understand the ladies, and that his education in the Arts of the Khama had been completed. Wood was even more incensed when he discovered that "Khama" meant "pleasure" and the Prince taunted him by saying that the Khama Sutra, which Wood described as "an unchaste oriental tract," might have been written for an innocent Englishman.

When Arthur left the harem he was fully recovered from his illness and dismissed Wood's suggestions that he should give evidence on "the happenings" to the American Mission. Wood's annoyance increased when Arthur treated the whole business with levity and showed an "uncalled for affection for the inmates." Although Lady Harriet had always shown a curiosity about life in a harem, Arthur did not mention his experiences in his letters and his diary records blandly, "Better, moved to Malichus Mirza's house for a change of air; and remained there till the 15th."(10)

Tom and Wood remained in Tabriz waiting for letters from Ireland, while Arthur set out alone for Mirza's country home. He rode seven hours each day, sleeping whenever he could; sometimes in sheds, sometimes in inns. On the 24th of January "nature was wearing her most disheartening aspect" - the landscape was covered in snow.(11) Joined by the others, he took a boat across Lake Umriah, sending the horses around by land. The boat was tossed about for six days in temperatures not rising above 15 degrees; they survived only because of their Russian furs and the Prince's arak. Wood was convinced that their privations were a punishment for Arthur's sins, and at the end of the journey the sport offered by the Prince was disappointing.

After a brief stay with American missionaries at Umriah, where the food was good but the temperance habit not greatly appreciated - it was cold weather

to be drinking cold water - they rode north into
Kurdistan. Their horses swam across swollen rivers;
their heavily laden mules fell into streams; they lay
down on the horse's backs to avoid the biting winds
and they stopped only when their mounts, struggling
up to their saddle-girths in snow drifts, refused to go
further. Some days ended with a "capital dinner" in the
house of a local official, others in cowsheds and once
when blinded with snow, they scooped out holes in the
drifts and slept in them. On the 24th February they
wrapped themselves in wolf skins and slept under their
horses for protection from an approaching storm. Arthur
appreciated the wildness and beauty of the scenery but
complained of pains in his chest, which he thought was
rheumatism. Even the censorious Wood was compelled
to praise his determination to take his fair share of
the hard tasks of their daily routine.

On the 9th March they rode into Mosul at sunset. Later
that month they awoke one morning to find themselves
locked in a courtyard; pistols were drawn and their
captors seemed to give way only when faced by a rider,
without arms or legs, wielding a gun. This at least was
Arthur's story to the Bruens, but in reality he felt they
were released because they had nothing worth stealing.

They descended the Tigris on rafts made of goat skins
and crossed the rapids at Nimrod on March 15th, when
Tom "shot a brace of partridge." On the 22nd March
Arthur recorded an encounter with a wild pig. "I got
a shot at a pig about fifty yards off but missed him
in a disgraceful manner." They arrived in Baghdad on
Arthur's birthday but rode off immediately into the
night to catch up with a party on its way to Babylon.
They met a strange caravan bringing bodies for burial at
the Holy City of Kerbola. Arthur dismissed the Tower
of Babel as a heap of burnt bricks, and less impressive
than the Pyramids; they returned to Baghdad on March
27th, disappointed.

Wood was not only at variance with Tom and Arthur
on the subject of their return home but also with Lady

Harriet. News of Arthur's poor health had reached
Borris and even produced a letter from Fanny Irvine:

"Newtown Park, February 26th 1850

"I hope dear Arthur, this will find you very much
improved in health and that you will very soon be
able to commence your journey homewards. We were
all sorry to hear you had been ill. Your mother,
Hoddy and Charley came here yesterday, all well
and in good spirits. Some of the young ladies beg
I would enclose a small flower of forget me not."

Lady Harriet, feeling the pain of sending Arthur away
and being anxious for him to come home, expected them
to turn back at Baghdad. Tom had written to Charley
telling him that he and Arthur were returning and he
welcomed the news. A letter written by Wood from
Tabriz had annoyed Lady Harriet by its vagueness; in
his reply to her he reminded her of the circumstances
in "which we quitted Ireland." Tom, he recalled,
was to travel for a year or two, but her instructions
regarding Arthur's "banishment" were that he should be
kept away from home for two or three years. She was
not reassured by the correspondence she received and
proposed that Arthur should return to Ireland to farm
land in Connemara, the bleak and ruggedly beautiful
part of Connacht, to which the less pliant Kavanaghs
had been transplanted by Cromwell two hundred years
earlier. Encouraged by Tom, Arthur accepted the plan.
"I would be exceedingly glad to undertake anything of
the sort that seemed at all likely to turn out well.
I think it suits my tastes better than taking a ready
made farm and having to pay rent which always went
against my grain." And so he resolved in the exile of
Connemara to be a source of comfort and assistance
to his mother rather than a "source of anxiety and
annoyance."(12)

While resting in Baghdad he entertained himself with
the "dancing boys" who were "a curious sight and not
over decent," and with a party of Italian girls.(13)
"Regina was certainly very handsome, not withstanding

a Baghdad button on her port cheek; a fine round stern, and well rigged aloft with a most luxurious pair of catheads. Rather course about the top gallan yards, she was a fine looking craft. Kemble junior (a member of the British Community) made fierce love to her, but as his main top mast did not reach her royals he looked more like her first cutter or launch than her consort." Although she had a most exceptional profile, Louisa "looked like a handsomely rigged schooner as she glided gracefully down the ballroom under the lee of the elder Kemble." However "her cats were not so fully developed as Regina's but firm enough to support any anchor she might ever want to hang there."

On April 23rd Arthur Tom and Wood joined members of the International Boundary Commission, then working in Persia, at the confluence of the Tigris and Karoum and travelled with them to spend Summer in the mountains. Between Bushir and Shiraz there were challenging ascents and descents. Cliff-like walls towered above and "worn out of solid rock is a narrow causeway, barely wide enough for a laden mule, with holes worn into regular steps like a cow track in soft ground, by the feet of thousands of beasts of burden . . . that have trodden it from ages past." Above was a sheer perpendicular wall of rock, "high enough almost to shut out the sight of day . . . " and "a sheer perpendicular precipice of rock below, losing itself in the shades of a dark and terrible abyss, and no parapet to save you from the effects of a single false step."

Arthur was feeling "as weak as a cat," deriving his strength from a daily dose of 16 grains of quinine. Normally he rode in the middle of the caravan with the horse's head tied to one of the baggage mules. On this ascent he decided to manage his own horse. It was lucky that he did because they were compelled to halt when "one of our number" became hysterical and refused to carry on. The man was taken from his horse and supported by two muleteers. The mule preceding Arthur, and to which his horse's head would normally have been tied, was awkwardly laden; one of the boxes it was carrying caught a rock and the shock staggered him. "I fancy I can see the unfortunate beast now and hear his cry of agony as he fell over the brink, the echo of the crash at the bottom being the last we ever heard of him or his load. It lasted but a minute, but in a second you can live an age; it would have been a relief to screech were it not for very shame; but the rear of the caravan pressed on behind and on I went filling up the gap in our ranks . . . "(14)

It was a wretched summer, a "hell upon earth." Arthur recorded temperatures of 120 degrees and the heat and glare intensified by the rock salt deposits brought down in the mountain streams making a salt desert "nearly roasted us alive." They found scorpions in Tom's bed and both Tom and Arthur suffered from fever and recurring headaches. Wood suffered from a throat infection and Arthur kept him company playing chess. They had read all their books and there was nothing to do but sleep and smoke. Sickness was frequent and one of their number died. Colonel Williams, head of the English group, to whom Arthur became attached, for he was "more like a father than a friend," was in charge of arrangements. They made "a rude coffin of store boxes and buried the man at noon in the valley, for only there was the soil deep enough." They wore "such black clothes as we happened to have." It was a melancholy funeral and threw gloom over the whole camp, leaving "a blank nothing can fill."(15)

On July 18th 1850 they turned north eastwards towards Baghdad and home. Arthur was keen to go via Tabriz, the home of Malichus Mirza, which made Wood suspicious and indignant. At Haroumabad Arthur got into a scrape with some gipsy girls. "Had great fun," he writes. The precise detail of the fun is uncertain for the relevant section of this page of his diary had been cut away. What remains reads "I thought it was all up with me but on raising my eyes and beholding the whole population grinning at my painfully ridiculous situation, shame got the better of lewdness, so imprinting one burning kiss (as Byron hath it) I escaped from her toils."(16)

- 63 -

Lady Harriet and Hoddy left for Corfu in June antici-
pating a reunion with Tom and Arthur later in the year.
They spent time in Albania on the way. The sea was
"perfectly smooth," the mountains magnificent and everywhere, writes Lady Harriet were "flocks of goats." They
ate hearty suppers from their own provisions and breakfasted on eggs and coffee bought in the villages, where
local men sat in a circle around them and watched them
eat "with the most tranquil gravity."(17) The privations
suffered by Lady Harriet and her daughter were mild
when compared to those suffered by Arthur and Tom,
although on the night of the 15th June they had no
toilet facilities and were compelled to lie down in their
clothes. In the morning they got up shaking themselves
"like dogs" before setting off again.

One of their party, a Mr Peacock, travelled with a
pistol in his belt for fear of robbers. Tempted by the
clear waters of a stream, he invited Lady Harriet to
go on ahead while he drank. "I had not proceeded ten
steps," she wrote, "when I heard the report of a pistol;
turning round I saw Mr Peacock stagger and fall at the
fountain - in stooping down, his pistol had gone off and
wounded him badly in the thigh."(18) It was a difficult
journey down to the town, with Mr Peacock in pain
and fainting on the back of a donkey. Though the heat
was "offensive" and the path took them "over rocks and
through tangled woods," Lady Harriet was not prevented
from noting the scenery as they went. Orchards and
cemeteries surrounded the town with it's "mosks and
minarets," and groves and "old castles backed up by
high blue mountains," and all "truly beautiful." Mr
Peacock recovered and Lady Harriet soon returned to
her sketching, expressing gratitude for the "liberty and
education with which Christians are blessed."(19)

There was no reunion in Corfu. In September Arthur
wrote, "I hope neither you, my dear mother, nor Hoddy
have suffered, in your useless trip to meet us, from
fevers prevalent in this horrid South."(20) Not only
fevers but lack of finance prevented them moving on.
Wood was sent to Baghdad to get money and Arthur

and Tom planned to meet him at Bushire and sail
for Ireland. During late Summer and Autumn their
movements are uncertain. They ran out of ink, and
the mixture of their own invention never dried, and
stuck pages together.

On the 23rd of December, Wood having returned with
money and, having failed in two attempts to travel
overland to India, they sailed, not for Ireland but for
Bombay. Only a double ration of grog distinguished
Christmas Day from any other as their ship proceeded
at a steady two and a half knots down the gulf, glad
to be leaving Persia behind them.

9. INDIA

Tom, Arthur and Wood, arrived in Bombay on January 5th 1851 and booked in at the Hope Hall Hotel. Tom and Wood involved themselves in a whirl of soirees and balls while Arthur busied himself with preparations for their journey inland. On Sunday Tom and Wood went to church; Arthur went to the horse dealers.

Wood had announced he was going to become "a great sportsman." "Heaven help the mark," Arthur commented. Wood's horse was an eight year old "brute", which had been "ridden by a lady and therefore suited him to a T," and he had "enough bullets to shoot all the tigers in India." What amused Arthur most was Wood's purchase of a boar spear " . . . his reason for which I could not make out as he seemed to find it difficult enough to sit on a horse without any such encumberance."(1)

Arthur meticulously listed their expenditure: a tent at 300 rupees; a pony and a buggy 300 rupees and a "well bred charger," 800 rupees. They set off for Poonah on the 20th January, Arthur riding "Sir John Grey." Fifteen "flunkies" and a cook in the buggy accompanied them. Within hours they had lost the buggy in a sea bog into which they had ridden in the darkness, and they had to wait for the moon to rise before they could find their path again.

Both Arthur and Wood described an encounter with a giant rat. Arthur simply writes "Had an encounter with a tremendous rat which I killed with Wood's spear."(2) Wood in describing the incident leaves us one of the few accounts of how Arthur used his stumps. " . . . he somehow succeeded in leaning over the horse's belly and with my boar spear between shoulders and stump impaled the huge rat in one swift movement - an amazing feat with so unwieldy and awkward a weapon."(3) Wood took Arthur's prowess for granted noting only the unwieldiness of the spear.

Each night the travellers showered, ate and slept in East India Company bungalows. Some were more comfortable than others; all were an improvement on their accommodation in Persia. What struck Arthur as "nonsense" was the etiquette so strictly observed by the British in India, which decreed that gentlemen who slept alongside one another did not speak because they had not been introduced.

As they moved on, the realisation that he was at last in India gave him much pleasure and he began to feel better in health. "The scenery was beautiful. The variegated foliage of the trees and the rich plumage of the paroquets and the humming birds as they flew screaming from tree to tree, made me realise that I was at length in the long awaited India."(4)

They arrived in Poonah on the 6th of February. Arthur noted without comment on the 9th, "Tom not feeling well." On the 20th they arrived in Aurungabad, which was to be their base for most of their stay in India.

They attended a review of the Nizam's Irregular Horse commanded by British officers, dined in the mess and interrogated the rope dancers through an interpreter. "A rope was thrown up into the air and one of the dancers caught it and seemed to soar up it until it was almost perpendicular, with himself at the top of it . . . I do not pretend to have found the answer to this; we questioned the dancer through an interpreter and could only gather it was done by some form of levitation peculiar to these people."(5) Arthur's happiness was complete when he persuaded his friend William Bookey's Commanding Officer to allow Bookey to join him on a shooting expedition.

Arthur shot his first tiger on March 29th from the back of an elephant. "Wood gave him one barrel which hit the ground close to his head, the only part of his body visible. I then took a pot shot at him and was fortunate enough to send my ball in behind his left ear." He was " . . . a fine young tiger, and quite nine feet

from tip of nose to end of tail."(6)   "The skin," Tom
wrote to Lady Harriet, "was adjudged to Arthur, who
hit him under the ear with his rifle, one of the most
effective shots."(7)   Tom further described how a tiger
leaped at the elephant Arthur was riding, tearing it's
trunk.   The "bag" for April 17th was "one cheetah and
two pigs;" for the 28th, "four tigers, one boar."   A
tiger "raised herself on her hind legs and commenced
growling and making faces at us when I sent a ball in
through her eye."(8)   Arthur recorded his less successful shots too.   "In the night three hyenas came to the
water to drink near my bed, I fired but the moon being
clouded, missed."(9)

When not complaining to Delhi about the continued
use of Temple prostitutes or deploring the "depressing
paraphernalia" of Hindu mysticism, Wood was writing
to Lady Harriet, telling her how difficult it was to
devise an itinerary.   "Your sons are such creatures of
impulse," and Arthur, he said, was motivated only by
what game was to be found.   "He says a tiger is better
worth seeing than ought else in India."   He "often
exposes himself to discomfort and fatigue in indulging
his passion for the chase, but I assure you he always
comes home from a hunting expedition in more robust
health, to all appearance, than when he started."(10)
Arthur was "not nearly so docile," wrote Tom, as when
ill in Persia, and would be inclined now to say, as the
criminal to the judge who sentenced him to transportation, "Thank you my Lord."(11)

In a quieter more reflective moment, Arthur wrote
"There are few things I enjoy more than, unseen to
watch the movements and habits of wild animals - to
see them as they are among themselves, pursuing their
various devices.   I have often lost a shot by thus
indulging my fancy and in no single instance did I ever
regret it".   "The variety of game one sees in the hot
season in India waiting through the night at a do or
pool, the only one perhaps within miles; each coming
in his own peculiar fashion; the timid deer - listening
for every sound - trying each breath of air for the

taint of an adversary; the sneaking hyena, the wolf and jackal with their slouching gate on the 'qui vive' alike for prey as for danger."(12)

Wood's references to Tom's health at this time indicated that he lacked Arthur's stamina; he told Lady Harriet that he was relieved that Tom showed less inclination to hunt than his brother. Tom and Wood spent long periods separated from Arthur and Bookey. Arthur considered that his brother and tutor "had done enough dancing," and wrote several letters trying to persuade them to join him. Tom usually replied that he would do so after the next ball, being more at home among the socialites than Arthur and Bookey. Arthur likened the mothers seeking husbands for their daughters, to man-eating spiders or to bazaar keepers setting out their wares, and the stiffness of life in fashionable Bombay had been one of the first things that disappointed him on arrival.

In June Tom haemorrhaged from the lungs. Lady Harriet was not aware of his condition, but was nevertheless vexed at her sons' prolonged absence and blamed Wood for it. If the purpose of the tour was to keep Arthur out of mischief it had clearly failed, particularly in Russia and Persia. Wood rejected Lady Harriet's criticism saying that he had urged Tom to return to Bombay to take the steamer before the monsoon season but, "Proposals, however, had been made by which the imagination of your sons was so greatly excited, that we should all join a great hunting party, and to these Tom listened."(13) Tom was again "unwell" and it was too late to get away before the monsoons. Feeling he had to justify his lack of control of the boys, one aged twenty three and the other twenty, Wood was ready, so he said, to quit. "I would on no account desire to remain longer in my present position than may seem necessary."(14)

When Tom and Arthur met to celebrate the news of the marriage of their sister Hoddy to Colonel Middleton, Arthur drank so much and laughed so much that he fell

off his chair which could not have pleased Wood, who
soon relieved himself of his post as Arthur's tutor. Tom
and Wood returned to Bombay in the Autumn of 1851,
leaving Arthur in Aurungabad. Tom, now suffering from
tuberculosis, was advised to return home via the Cape
or through the Mediterranean to take advantage of the
rest and the warm sea breezes. The advice was ignored,
and on December 8th they sailed for Java en route for
Adelaide. Wood justified his actions by saying that
Arthur was capable of looking after himself and Tom
was more in need of his care.

They had, Arthur said, left him in "a bit of a fix."
Half of the 400 rupees Tom had given him before his
departure was spent on paying his debts, leaving him
about eleven pounds to live on. Bookey was back with
his regiment and Arthur was alone in India. He wrote
to his mother asking her to send two hundred pounds
so that he could return home via Greece, leaving Tom
and Wood to return "round the other side of the globe."

There was no swift reply from Lady Harriet, and under
a cheerful exterior Arthur lived, initially, a "wretched
existence." He didn't discuss his finances with his
compatriots but one of them, Mrs Penruddock, sensed
his concern at the absence of news of his family, and
discovered that he was limiting himself to one meal
a day. She described him: "A wonderful horseman,
he spent most of his time riding, though he could hop
about on his stumps with astonishing agility. He made
great friends with the native children and often used
to sit under a tree in the garden, painting them as they
sat in wonderment at this surprising man who held a
brush so dexterously between his two stumps."(15)

He used his skill as a horseman to earn his living,
carrying despatches in the Aurungabad district, and
undertook long and arduous rides. During one of these
his diary for this period was lost in a flooded river.
His offer to travel to Persia to report on Russian
intentions there was declined by the Government and
he obtained instead a report on the situation from

Malichus Mirza. He readily gave his opinions on how
Britain should deal with Russia - by seizing the Punjab
and holding on to the mountainous regions - and foresaw
that British insensitiveness could lead to India becoming
as troublesome as Ireland.

Eventually he gave up despatch riding and took a clerical
post in the Survey Department of the Poonah district,
with a salary of four hundred pounds annually. His dress,
despite his relative poverty, was "immaculate." There
was never a wrinkle in his tunic and he wore his topi
and his white satin cloak with the air of a man born to
wear good clothes. Mrs Penruddock found him handsome,
virile and authoritative. "He wanted to please everybody
and this applied equally to Indians and Europeans. I
remember that he was particularly surprised that there
should be no word in Hindi or Urdu for 'thank you!'
We had never before realised this omission and it just
hadn't occurred to us to seek for any such phrase."
Arthur chose as an alternative, "sweetness be upon
your life," which Mrs Penruddock, less courteous and
sensitive in her dealings with the Indians, considered
"sugary" and wasted upon "totally illiterate people."(16)

In February 1852 Arthur received a letter from Wood
telling him Tom was better, but expressing anxiety about
both Tom's and Arthur's sinfulness. Although deploring
Tom's long estrangement from his Saviour, Wood believed
that Tom's illness was a blessing, but warned Arthur
that no such time for repentance would necessarily be
given to him. In June 1852 Lady Harriet wrote to Tom,
addressing her letter to Adelaide. Influenced by Wood,
she urged him to place his trust in Christ his Saviour,
"who pleads for you in heaven."(17) Like Arthur, she
was unaware that Tom was already dead.

Lady Harriet set out for Corfu in July to visit Hoddy
and her husband, whose regiment was stationed there.
Arthur left India at about the same time, carried on
board ship by a servant who accompanied him on part
of the journey. One of his last purchases in India was
a small filigree box which he said enigmatically was "for
my wife."

There was no definite news of Tom until on the 21st August the black-edged columns of the Carlow Sentinel announced the death of "Thomas Kavanagh Esquire on a passage from Sumatra to Australia for the benefit of his health." In the usual platitudes they spoke of Tom as lamented by his family and tenantry, "to whom he was so strongly attached." His conduct since his coming of age, they saw, as evidence of his intention to follow in his father's footsteps as one of "the best and most munificent of landlords and country gentleman."(18) The truth was that Tom was rarely in Ireland and scarcely known to his tenants. The news of his death some five months earlier, followed by his burial at sea, came in a longwinded letter from Wood to Lady Harriet. At first he had been unable to bring himself to write, and when he did so he found difficulty in coming to the point. The news of Tom's death was followed soon by the news of Wood's own death in unexplained circumstances.

Tom was succeeded on "his extensive estates by his brother Charles Kavanagh, late of the 7th Hussars," and Arthur was his heir. The 'Legend' had been fulfilled.(19) Early in 1853 plans for Charles' marriage the following Easter were announced. It would be a marriage which challenged Arthur's position as heir to the Kavanagh Estates and also 'The Legend'. However on the morning of the 20th February, Charles, shaving in his room, was standing "too near to the fireplace," and "his morning robe caught fire and blazed about him." In attempting to put out the flames he threw himself on his bed, but his burning clothes set light to the covers and bed-curtains and he was "fearfully burned in many parts of his body." (20) Boxwell and two of his colleagues rushed to Borris House, but Charles' burns were too severe for there to be any hope of recovery, and he died the following day. Charles had suffered all his life from "little attacks," which may have been a mild form of epilepsy, and he may well have fallen into the fire. Arthur, who had been so badly received on the day of his birth, was now Master of Borris.

10.   MASTER OF BORRIS

From Borris as far as the eye could see in any direction
was Kavanagh land.   An estimated 30,000 acres, it was
not among the largest of Irish estates but large enough
to sustain the family's privileged life style.

During Tom's long minority the Kavanaghs had become
absentee landlords, like so many of the Protestant
Ascendancy which Thomas Kavanagh had joined to
sustain the family's power and influence.   While the
Irish starved, the Kavanagh boys drank champagne and
ate caviar in Moscow; while Father John Walshe
complained that "to send enfeebled old age, clothed in
looped garments to stand in water amid the frosts
of winter for 7d a day, is such treatment of a fellow
creature I can never sanction,"(1)   Charles Kavanagh
was attending Levees in Dublin Castle, in a presence
chamber newly hung with crimson silk, before a throne
covered with crimson velvet and dominated by the
Royal Arms raised in tapestry of gold and silver
"of the most exquisite taste."(2)

For the first time in their history the Kavanaghs were
separated, by their new allegiances, from their people.
Lady Harriet was the vehicle of the "unhappy connection"
with the myriads of the English Prime Minister Pitt, who
had destroyed the Irish Parliament to no good purpose.(3)
Periodically she had returned to Borris with her children
to be feted like a sovereign, to hear speeches about the
bonds between landlords and the soil and to receive
loyal toasts from a well fed and fork-tongued tenantry,
before disappearing again to bask in the sun of the
Mediterranean and beyond.   At least that is how it
seemed to those left behind.

During the fifteen years of the "minority," Doyne had
administered the estates. He was a hard man and a good
manager, intent on introducing new farming techniques.
However the tenants felt no loyalty to him and resented

him as the "middle man." Lady Harriet was suspect and even hated by some. Tom had never honoured his promises to live amongst them once he had reached his majority, and Charles was an enigmatic Hussar who suffered from "little attacks" and whose terrible death confirmed that the family was cursed.

Arthur, the determined, courageous, dare-devil cripple, who was now Master of Borris against all odds, resolved to clear the family's name, and restore its standing to what he imagined it had been during his father's time. He would, he thought, be as good a landlord and as active a Parliamentarian as his father. He knew the tenants, and they had known him from his unhappy birth. As a teenager he had lectured them at Harvest Homes, on the bonds he felt he had with them, on their common heritage and on how to make bread from the tainted potato crop. Like them he seemed deserted by the family, and like many of their kin he had been banished. These shared experiences, and his strength, charm and affection, and his streak of "the wild colonial boy," appealed to them.

In 1853 he became "under-agent" on the Borris estates and a serious student of estate management. The famine had defeated the efforts of landlords and tenants to improve their property and holdings. There was no rent to be had from a physically and financially exhausted tenantry; land went unworked, and this, along with the tumble-down cottages and ruined thatch, gave the country-side an air of desolation. Just as Lady Harriet's father had transformed Balinasloe from a slum into a pleasant place to live, so Arthur decided to transform his estates. He combined the energy, reorganising ability and public spiritedness of the le Poer Trenches with the generosity, warmth and religious tolerance of his father. Before he began to put his plans into operation there were domestic matters to be dealt with and old friendships to be renewed. Lady Harriet's courage failed her when sorting Tom's papers. She re-read the letter about the "fateful" game of billiards with Wood, the outcome of which had determined that Tom would travel on to India rather than return home; being unable to continue, she handed the task to Arthur. Wood's next of kin wrote asking for money, which they claimed was due to Wood at the time of his death in Australia. Arthur was businesslike and firm. In refusing their request, he told them Wood had been provided with ample money for his needs and was owed nothing.

As Boxwell and Lady Harriet had planned in the early years, Arthur had become oblivious to his defects and "no one who came across him was five minutes in his company without forgetting all his peculiarities."(3) His horsemanship, which was taken for granted, enabled him to get around the estate, while elsewhere he was carried on the back of a body servant, whose existence he and everyone else seemed to ignore. Sometimes he was carried in a basket; but the indignity of all this was obliterated by the power of his presence.

In the House he received visitors seated and wearing a cloak. When he felt he wanted to get closer to them he slid down from the chair and "hopped" - a term he disliked - or propelled himself across the room. He wrote with a pen between his stumps or attached to a hook, and in estate cottages tenants looked on amazed when he signed receipts with a pen between his teeth.(4)

In September 1853 he acted as a steward for the first time at Carlow races. In the "green refreshing warmth" of June 1854 he returned to Celbridge for the wedding of his childhood friend Mary Conolly. It was a quiet family affair in the village church. The Duke of Leinster, The Marquis and Marchioness of Headford, Lady Harriet Kavanagh and Arthur Kavanagh Esq headed the guest list of eighty persons who sat down at Castletown for a "sumptuous dejeuner" of every delicacy the season could afford."(5)

In the Autumn of 1854 "an interesting event came off," when eighty tenants dined at Borris to celebrate the Harvest. It was a modest gathering compared with those of the past but the food was still plentiful, as was the

supply of "seasonable liqueurs."(6) Fanny Irvine, to
whom he had referred rashly as his "dearest wife", was
not among the guests, having been replaced by Frances
Leathly, the daughter of a clergyman from Louth. She
was a distant cousin, being the granddaughter of Lady
Harriet Osborne, Arthur's great aunt on his mother's
side.

"She had a sweet, almost submissive disposition but
this was deceptive," says Sarah Steele. "Though shy
and sometimes embarrassingly modest, she hid beneath
a docile exterior a tremendous strength of character."
"She had known Arthur since she was a child and had
admired intensely his wonderful exploits. We always
thought it was Lady Harriet herself who determined
that Frances would make an ideal wife for Arthur.
Frances had been a favourite of hers from childhood."
(7) As the new year dawned Boxwell, still prepared
to wager on a birth despite the outcome of his wager
with Thomas twenty three years earlier, let it be
known that he was putting his money on there being
an heir in Borris House within a year.

Arthur married Frances Leathly on the 15th March
1855 in the drawing room of his Aunt Louisa's house,
No 1 Mountjoy Square, Dublin. It is an elegant orange
brick Georgian house standing on a rise to the North
of the city. The vicar of Clongoose officiated - the
Kavanagh chapel at Borris House served as the Parish
Church of Clongoose.

The ceremony in Dublin was "quiet" but the celebrations
in Borris were held "on a scale seldom witnessed."(8)
The financial problems of the previous year appeared to
be forgotten, and from the early hours of March 27th
the tenants began to arrive. First came those from
St Mullins with their wives and children in their "best
attire," followed by those from Ballyragget. Arthur met
them at the gates and, preceded by a band, led them
to the house where they saw "the graceful form of
the future mistress of Borris." The "fair daughter of
Louth," accompanied by her mother-in-law and her

aunt, "the ugly and obliging daughters" of the late Earl
of Clancarty, received a truly "Celtic Welcome."

It was a fine day and the tables were set out in the
Courtyard under awnings topped with Union Jacks and
Tricolours, much as they had been in better years.
Arthur and Frances sat at the head of a table heavy
with barons of beef "of enormous magnitude," flitches
of bacon, ham, roast beef, mutton, salmon from the
River Barrow, and plum cakes. Ale and wine flowed
freely. After dinner at 4 pm Moses Leach proposed
a long-winded toast, more to his own unworthiness
than to the happiness of the bride or groom, and was
interrupted by cries of "Long life to Mr Kavanagh,"
and "Long may he reign over us." There was "good
feeling" all around, Arthur was happy to be home at
"dear Borris" and the tenantry were pleased by the
prospect of having a landlord once more living among
them. The toast to Lady Harriet was interrupted by
a cry of "may she be the happy grandmother of many
grandchildren," and the band played the Air St Patrick.
At dusk bonfires glowed on Mount Leinster and along the
Blackstairs range, and "the multitude," which included
Bookey home from India, "danced to the violins."(9)

Dynastically it was a poor match. Unlike Lady Harriet
and the aristocratic Ormonde women, Frances brought
no addition to the Kavanagh lands and no influential
ties, but Arthur was in love with her and she "admired
his exploits."(10) What the private thoughts of the
sweet, submissive and modest maid from Louth were,
as she entered her marriage to the handsome, dare-
devil "cripple" schooled in the arts of Khama, are not
known; but within a month she was pregnant.

In his twenty fifth year Arthur was the owner of estates
with great potential wealth, Chairman of his local Bench
of Magistrates, a lively socialite, sportsman, husband,
and father-to-be.

On the Borris estates he remitted rents outstanding since
Doyne's agency and as leases ended renewed them, often

at a nominal rent. He rebuilt, re-roofed and redesigned
the houses in the villages and his design for the best
slate-roofed cottage, at the lowest cost, won him the
medal of the Dublin Society.

In Ballyragget the Georgian Lodge, with its splendid
staircase and perfectly proportioned rooms, became Lady
Harriet's home. It stood on the banks of the Nore among
beech, lime and ilex and in the shadow of the ruined
castle which had once been the home of Anne Boleyn.
Bookey acted as Arthur's agent here and the village was
transformed into a well ordered pleasant place to live.
Timber and slate were supplied free to those tenants
willing to improve their holdings. Feelings towards the
landlord and his agent were generous and when Bookey's
corn was in need of securing, the townsfolk marched out
to help him, returning behind a band to drink and dance
into the night and toast the health of "Arthur Kavanagh
and his amiable lady."(11)

He sat regularly as chairman of the Borris Magistrates
with Blackney, whose family had ousted his father
from Parliament, and Sweetman who had provoked a
public enquiry into allegations of mismanagement on the
Kavanagh estates at St Mullins. He committed Michael
Somers to the Quarter Sessions for assault on Margaret
Doyle on the Feast of the Assumption and adjudicated in
the case of Sarah and John Curran who, returning from
a local fair, had beaten John Doyle unmercifully with a
stick so that, according to Dr Boxwell's testimony, he
took to his bed for sixteen days. He adjudicated when
Joseph Dalton, Anne Doyle and others were convicted
of theft of boughs from the Borris estate, and were
fined two shillings.

On the 14th January 1856 at 3.30 in the afternoon,
Frances gave birth to a son, whom they called Walter.
Every dwelling in the village was illuminated "with
various devices tastefully suited for the occasion."
Tar barrels blazed in the streets, and fires glowed
in the mountains. The solitary bell of the Catholic
Chapel rang and the parish priest's house resembled

"a fairy palace." To one anonymous onlooker it was
one of the most stirring events that had occurred for
many years in the history of Borris. With a note of
caution he rejoiced that "an heir is come forth to
inherit, please providence, the Kavanagh's properties;
and while I write the town is all enthusiasm - the
cheers of delighted thousands greet my ears - the town
is brilliantly illuminated in every direction and the
surrounding mountains are lit up with bonfires." A
stray bonfire was observed even in far away Kilkenny,
and Arthur was described as a "generous landlord,
anxious to promote social progress and the happiness
of his people. He is no racketeer. He gives the land
for fair value and wishes to see even the poorest of
his estates happy."(12)

At 7 pm Arthur, a superb figure on horseback, with a
cloak falling in folds from his broad shoulders disguising
his limblessness, rode to the gates of Borris House
to watch the festivities and to receive the tenants
congratulations.

It was a good year. He was elected by his peers to
the Grand Jury - the forerunner of the County Council -
and nominated High Sheriff in Kilkenny. In the Autumn,
when a smaller number than usual sat down to celebrate
the Harvest, Frances announced her plans to supplement
the savings of each villager with a gift of her own.
She was again pregnant.

11.   DIARIES 1857

Arthur's diaries for the years 1857-1860 have survived.
They are small Almanacs crammed with facts and figures,
weights and measures and important dates in the Civil
and Ecclesiastical calendar. He used either Chambers
Pocket Almanac or The Pocket Book published by Punch.
With a week to a page, the entries are inevitably brief,
giving a glimpse of his daily life and listing, usually at
the end, the "high lights" of the year. In 1857 he singled
out the illness of his elder son Walter, the birth of his
his second son Arthur, his appointment as High Sheriff
in Carlow, and his mother's departure for India.

February 4th was "an unseasonably hot day" and "baby
got sick."(1)   Arthur and Frances were alarmed, and
the following day Frances consulted their old friend
Sir Philip Crampton. Frances wrote from Dublin, and
Arthur recorded "letter from Fan, baby's case more
serious than we had hoped".(2) There were no details
of the illness and its nature remained uncertain, but
Frances was distressed and Arthur wrote her a gentle
consoling letter which reveals his own philosophy.

"I am very sorry my own dearest that you should write
in so sad a mood. The dreadful anxiety completely
knocked me down. It is very hard to place one's whole
trust and confidence in God. I do not think the trust
you should try to feel is that God will avert anything,
but to trust implicitly that what He orders is for the
best; to feel that He is your oldest, dearest, firmest
friend; that when you are in trouble you can, as it
were, put your hand out, and lean on His Almighty
arm - sure that He is both able and willing to help
you in every time of need. This alone can take the
sting from earthly sorrow; but it does take it indeed!
Had I not felt it, I would not say so. So try to feel
it, dearest Fuz - feel that Walter has a Father in Him
who watches over him day and night, and without

whose leave a hair of his head cannot fall. Trust him implicitly in His mercy."

"Do not think that I am canting or that what I say is hypocrisy. Inconsistent as I am, I do feel in my heart that God hears my prayers. I have often been startled at their being so quickly answered, and sometimes so literally. I try to pray for every little thing that I want, and when sometimes the thing came, or happened unexpectedly - trivial as it might be - I could not help thinking that it was sent as an encouragement."

"One of the greatest comforts is to feel that God sees every thought of one's heart. He knows the frailty of one's nature, and in His mercy forgives the bad, while the faintest shortest prayer breathed, or even felt in the heart, is seen also - seldom though it be. I cannot express exactly what I mean, but I often feel that it is so, and I think that the feeling increases one's trust in God. The 'dreadful anxiety' was almost unbearable until that feeling of trust began to come again, and, as I prayed, it strengthened until I believed that in His never failing mercy He had again heard me. I still think and believe He has - for Jesus Christ's sake. 'Whatsoever thou shalt ask in My name I will give it,' is a promise, although centuries old, as strong and sure as the day it was made. I don't want to preach dearest but I do sometimes feel what I have written - too seldom indeed. Inconsistent proud, often dissatisfied with what I deem a monotonous life, often forgetful of God, I still feel he came not to call the righteous, but sinners in repentance."(3)

Like his mother at his own birth, he accepted adversity as being "for the best", not in a negative fatalistic sense, but in the belief that no real harm could come about and much that is positive be drawn out of a situation. There was an almost childlike dependence on the "Heavenly Father" and an acknowledgement that he himself fell short of living up to his ideals. The dissatisfaction with his own temper, his arrogance and the other frailties of "our nature" were never far from the surface. Arthur was not well enough to attend the Spring Assizes, but on his birthday was present as High Sheriff for the proclamation of the election in the borough of Carlow. There was some cynicism among the electorate due to Sadlier, a previous member, having been a "placeman." He had made wild promises to the voters only to abandon his constituency once he had become a Junior Lord of the Treasury under Lord Aberdeen. He was the Mr Meddle of Dicken's 'Little Dorrit' and after bringing disaster to small farmers in the South of Ireland through his financial chicanery had been found dead on Hampstead Heath with a silver cream jug and several bottles of poison beside him. Arthur's candidate was the less colourful Mr Alexander who was engaged to his niece.

An "imposing force of cavalry," as well as infantry and police, were lined up outside the Court House for Arthur's arrival but there was, says the Carlow Sentinel, "little excitement." Arthur took his seat at 10 am and the election was proclaimed by his Deputy. The meeting was turbulent but good humoured. Any mention of Sadlier brought groans and hisses or a few provocative cheers. Arthur presided good naturedly over the laughter and the ribaldry, interspersed with cries of "Well done old cock." (4) Alexander's speech was modest, almost sanctimonious. He told his listeners how much he would prefer life at home with his family, but public duty had led him to stand. The electors liked him and on April 2nd Arthur records briefly, "Went into Carlow at 10 am and opened Court. Alex returned by 43 votes."(5)

As the clock struck three on the morning of the 27th August a watchful Arthur noticed a light in Fan's room and got up to investigate. She was in labour. He roused Bowers, one of the servants whose impertinence he found unbearable, and sent him for the midwife while he sat down to write a letter to one of his Kilkenny cousins asking him not to come to breakfast. In his diary he wrote "Youngster born at half past four."(6)

Frances quickly recovered from her confinement, and Arthur delighted in driving her out in the pony carriage, the reins lashed around and between his stumps. Sometimes they collected rents together. In October they went on a short winter cruise prescribed by Sir William Jenner for young Walter's health, which seemed to get no worse.

In November 1857, after weeks of preparation, Lady Harriet and Hoddy left for India: "November 24th, Mother and Hod started by the early train on route for India."(7) Arthur had carefully listed times of departure from Southampton and Marseilles, helped with their financial arrangements and generally supervised their preparation. When, in the Spring of the next year, he recorded, "Mother's Calcutta bill came through," the tables were reversed from earlier times when it was Lady Harriet who was receiving a succession of bills and pleas for money from Tom and Arthur.

Arthur enjoyed hunting. He rode frequently with his Butler relatives at Gowran Castle, a grey house in parkland over the river Barrow in Kilkenny. His courage as a rider was admired by them all and they often stopped, breathless, until he had taken a fence safely. He was however as much an object of horror as admiration, and in the drawing room one morning a child screamed with fear when she saw him - "a man sitting on the sideboard - well not a man - a torso in a pink coat."(8) The child, rooted to the spot, shrieked and shrieked until her mother, who was still fastening her riding habit, rescued her. Unable to speak, she pointed at Arthur and was quietly led away by an admonishing parent.

She later claimed that her fear was not so much due to Arthur's physical disabilities as to his being the cripple of the legend and a representative of those who had brought the Normans into Ireland. The story had recently been portrayed in Daniel Maclise's gigantic painting of the Kavanagh, King of Leinster, MacMurrough presenting his daughter, the Princess Eva, in marriage to Strongbow the Norman leader, while "disconsolate figures strewn in the foreground symbolised the destruction of the old Gaelic society."(9)

Bookey and Arthur's Pakenham relatives were frequent visitors to Borris, often arriving for breakfast prior to a day of duck shooting. The Boxwells were frequent guests at dinner, but when Florinda Bookey came they were all obliged to eat by candle light as she could not tolerate the newly installed gas lighting. At dinner Arthur served himself to soup, though it is uncertain whether he did this with the help of a hook attached to his stumps or with a ladle held between his stumps. The American poet Richard Hovey does not enlighten us in his glimpse of supper at Borris.

> "A stone jug and a pewter mug,
> And a table set for three,
> A jug and a mug in every place
> And a biscuit or two with Brie!
> Three stone jugs of Cruiskeen Lawn,
> And a cheese like custard foam "
> The Kavanagh receives tonight
> MacMurrough is at home.(10)

Arthur was happy entertaining and being entertained. When Lawrence Alexander married Harriet Bruen, his niece, in June 1857, there were 40 guests at Borris for the wedding breakfast. With the Conollys, Pakenhams and Bookeys, Arthur and Frances headed the guest lists at the balls at Oak Park, but many days were monotonous with tedious hearings on the Bench and patient listening to tenants complaints beneath the old oak tree in the Courtyard, as his father had done, wrapped in his cloak and smoking a cigar. At the Ross Poor House he was obliged to listen to Father Doyle's complaints against the doctor. He often felt "seedy" and suffered from "tooth-ache," but two bulls home successfully from a show compensated and if he was short of money Frances would always oblige: "borrowed 4/- from Fan."(11)

12. DIARIES 1858-9

After five years the gloss on being a country gentleman was wearing thin. The early days of 1858 were decidedly monotonous: "Went to church, got seedy, nervous from smoking."(1)   Sometimes while others went to church Arthur stole away to the top of the hill and sat reading or, with a sense of guilt, "dawdled in the drawing room till tiffin."(2)   Some cold days the ride to Ballyragget was fruitless; there was "no rent to be had,"(3) and the effects of the Famine were still being felt in the country which had lost half its population. Frances' friends could be tedious and Mrs Barrington and Mrs Stoppard were two he could not put up with.   When they came he "bolted" and "went axing."(4)

Most tedious of all were the committees which involved him in endless discussions of trivialities, such as the application of a Carlow doctor to the Board of Guardians for an increased fee for attendance outside his area. The doctor put his case, aided by sketch maps showing the distances walked; "a long and desultory conversation then ensued." Finally as if in desperation, Mr Newton, one of Arthur's neighbours, proposed the fee be given. Arthur seconded this with rapidity and the doctor got his fee.(5)

If there were difficult days there were also sleepless nights. Arthur and Frances were not distant Victorian parents and when young Walter got croup, it was Arthur who called Boxwell and remained up until 2 am until he was assured the boy was alright.

He hunted regularly with Denis Pack-Beresford, a former High Sheriff, whose father was the first and last Viscount Beresford, illegitimate son of The Marquis of Waterford; and with the Conollys and Bruens. But more and more he sought solace in "axing." He could wield an axe between his stumps and often, at this period, felled trees in his favourite spot, near the ruined chapel at Ballycoppigan, until Frances brought him tea which they took within the sound of the rushing waters of the brook. On the way back they savoured the views of the House, majestic in the distance. On St George's day he "axed beech tree, got it down in two hours with another."(6) The "other" was often Boxwell, and one day he records how they cut down five trees between them.

In 1858 he bought the hull of a vessel, the 'Triumvir', which was lengthened, fitted out and rigged as a schooner. He found the name ugly and re-christened her 'Corsair'. She was moored at Ross, within easy distance of Borris, and became a means of escape from the damp Irish weather, the tedium of long hours on the Bench and the paltry matters before the Grand Jury or the Board of Guardians.

In May, Arthur was in London, in a flurry of activity buying watches and charts at Fortnum and Mason, hurrying by train from Waterloo to Lymington in order to supervise the loading of stores and fitting of tanks before setting sail on Corsair, only to be becalmed off Calshott.

The sea freed him from the day to day demands of an Irish landlord, and left him space for reflection sometimes tinged with regret. On May 22nd, alone in his cabin, he wrote in his diary:

> "Man your equal weak as you, not fit to be your judge may well be shut out from the secrets of your heart; as for what lies below leave that to God. But take it to your Maker, show him the secrets of your spirit. He gave, ask Him how you are to bear the pain he has appointed. Kneel in his presence, pray with Faith for light in darkness for strength in weakness."(7)

His family and friends understood little of his secret life: his pain at what he was; the darkness and the weakness. His wife, like his mother, never alluded to his disabilities. For her they did not exist, and the most she could do was to admire him. His charm and liveliness made it all seem easy to them. In the writing of letters, the wielding of an axe, the handling of a soup ladle, the holding of reins, he enabled others to forget the effort needed for each move.

In the Summer, Frances took a house in Dunmore and was near to Arthur on his trips to Ross. On May 29th the Carlow Sentinel reported that "Corsair, 150 tons belonging to Mr Arthur Kavanagh of Borris House put into Dunmore East on Friday evening last with Mr and Mrs Kavanagh, their family and suite on board." "The Corsair, bound for a Summer trip up the Mediterranean to Corfu, was compelled to run into Dunmore to await a more favourable wind and the Corsair yet remains alongside."

The Kavanaghs spent June cruising in the Eastern Mediterranean and returned to Borris in time for church on the 27th. After a visit to Dublin on the 28th of June and the lancing of a boil in his nose on the 29th, he was off to Ross and Corsair again on the 9th July. On the 10th he anchored off Queenstown. On the 22nd July he was in Kingstown harbour. "Just as we were sitting down to breakfast, mother arrived having landed at 5 am from Liverpool."(8) Undaunted by her long return journey from India, Lady Harriet spent the day in Dublin with Arthur.

He was delighted when he was elected a member of the Royal Yacht Squadron and saddened by the death of his friend from childhood, Sir Philip Crampton. Like so many others, in the words of the Sentinel he was "deprived of a source to which we feel accustomed to look."(9)

At the beginning of August the Kavanaghs sailed for Cherbourg for the Queen's visit to Emperor Napoleon III. The Queen had had a rough passage but she was not ill and received the Emperor on board. "An electric light was thrown on the Emperor's barge following it the whole way up the harbour," and the Queen went below and "nearly finished that most interesting book Jane Eyre," while Arthur, Lady Harriet and Bookey went to see the illuminations. The following day "The harbour was literally swarming with craft brave with gala array and there was a firework display costing 2500 francs.(10)

In September Arthur was back in Borris hunting before breakfast, drawing the first bow in the archery contests at Gowran, with the aid of a hook, and driving with Fan in the afternoons. His duties as a magistrate, Poor Law Guardian and landlord no longer merited a mention. In September he gave up smoking and wondered "how long will it last ?"(11)

As Christmas 1858 approached he was in a reflective mood, meditating on the 51st psalm.

"Be gracious to me O God, in thy true love
In the fulness of thy mercy blot out my misdeeds,
Wash away all my guilt
and cleanse me from my sin.
For well I know my misdeeds
and my sins confront me all the day long."

Of more significance in the 51st psalm are the words

"In iniquity I was brought to birth
and my mother conceived me in sin;
yet, though thou has hidden the truth in darkness
through this mystery thou dost teach me wisdom."(12)

This is perhaps the nearest Arthur could come to an explanation of his deformities, a punishment for sin, his own yet uncommitted, or for those of others. Such feelings of guilt and sin were a part of the evangelical tradition at this period. He frequently accused himself of arrogance, and bad temper, but twentieth century gossip or lore have chosen to interpret "sin" as a sexual matter. Building on Arthur's adolescent exploits during the Smith O'Brien period, his introduction to the Arts of Khama in Malichus Mirza's harem and his lewd episode with the gipsies in Haroumabad, local gossip and lore hint at a range of extra marital affairs with local girls, and although this is repeated and often accepted, no evidence is produced for these assertions, which seem based on little more than the popular belief that every landlord exercised his "seignorial rights."

Arthur certainly had a pre-occupation with the love lives of his visitors and neighbours. In his 1857 diary he had drawn a broken heart in the margin beside an entry saying "poor Vernon driven to the train - lovers lost in the wood;"(13) and in his 1859 diary, "Went out with Moses for a stroll and heard confession and state of his feelings." A little later, "noticed lovers on stone bridge during morning ride, fancied Moses case looked hopeful, bet £4 on it" and finally "went out with disappointed lovers, lively walk, poor little Moses went by the late train, much to be pitied, 'faint heart,'"(14)

In addition to the usual activities at Christmas, with Arthur supervising the cutting of joints to be given as gifts to the poor, the parcelling of blankets and flannel, which he delivered himself, riding to remote farms and cabins, there was the grand event of the extension of the railway line to Borris. The enterprise, which was under the supervision of a Mr Mott, an Englishman, ran into financial difficulties. Having donated a strip of land fourteen miles in length for the track from Bagnelstown, Arthur took over the project, which transformed the valley with the construction of a viaduct. He put in £5000 to hold the operation until it was taken over by the local Railway Company. The line was opened on Christmas Day, while a week before the press carried a letter of complaint about the inappropriate timing of connections with Kilkenny.

On Christmas morning Frances was "too seedy" to come to breakfast. In the afternoon Arthur, Frances, Bess Pakenham and the Trenches drove to Mount Leinster. In the evening children from the village sang carols on the grand staircase, to the family seated in the hall; everyone was given a present except the footmen and cook "for reasons best known to themselves."(15)

On Boxing Day Frances was still "seedy," and Arthur
sat up with her and "smoked." His intention of giving
up smoking in September had not lasted and the year
ended with the worried husband consulting Boxwell
about Frances' health.

With the beginning of 1859 Arthur's thoughts on the
inscrutability of God's ways surfaced again. In a
contemplative vein he wrote,

> "When is the time for prayer?
> In every hour while life is spared
> In crowds in solitude to thee in joy in care
> Thy thoughts should heavenward flee."

and he notes the Book of Isaiah, Chapter 55, "verse 6
to the end,"(16) which reminds the reader " . . . my
thoughts are not your thoughts and your ways are not
my ways." For Arthur, longing for things to be different,
there was consolation in the belief that all things were
ordered for a purpose.

Piety and opulence combined easily in him and he was
at the new year party at Gowran Castle where, as was
usual, the dancing went on into the night. It was a
"great supper and very jolly party," but when they arrived
at Borris at 3 am the gates were closed against them
and the cantankerous gate-keeper Commons, who rivalled
Bowers in impertinence, nowhere to be found. They failed
"with every device" to attract his attention and eventually
Moses Leach, one of the party, scaled the demesne wall
and found Commons eating bread and cheese in the gate
house. It was 5 am before they "turned in." The day
was foggy and Arthur "settled accounts" and "went about
the demesne with the ladies."(17) Arthur records two
of their guests, Charley and Bill, as going back to the
yacht. These two may have been Lord Charles and Lord
William Beresford, sons of the Marquis of Waterford.
Charles was a teenager and keen sailor and became one
of Arthur's life long friends. The Beresford boys, noted
for their wildness, once rode a pig down Picadilly and a
horse up the stairs to their mother's bedroom. They
were kinsmen of the bachelor Dennis Pack-Beresford,

who frequently breakfasted at Borris before a day's shooting with Arthur.

The entries in his diary began to look alike. "Fine mild morning shooting with G Pakenham, T Bookey, Moses and self - 24 pheasants, 5 woodcocks, 7 rabbits . . . "(18) In the evenings the friends played bagatelle in the hall.

One February morning Arthur and Bookey went to Matins at St Mullins in the little chapel alongside the Kavanagh burial ground. In the vault beneath lay his father, his brother Charles and his half sister Mary Wandsford, who was married and dead by the age of fourteen. Outside in the graveyard lay Art Kavanagh, King of Leinster, poisoned at Ross in 1417, and the remains of the cell of St Moling. This hallowed spot did not dampen their high spirits and walking down to the small quay, Bookey "fell in river and wet himself." (19)

At the meeting of the poor Law Guardians on the 11th of January there had been an acrimonious discussion of Boxwell's salary. That he and Arthur had played a game of bagatelle the previous evening could not have harmed the doctor's case. Arthur argued that while it was their duty "to keep down the expenses as much as possible, it also devolves upon us to provide a proper medical man to attend to the wants of the poor. Of course persons in affluent circumstances always secure a first class doctor when they require him, but it is not so with the poor. If you do not give a liberal salary you cannot expect a proper officer."(20)

Two members of the Board disputed Boxwell's need for a second horse, implying that the beast was not kept for his rounds but so that he could follow the Kilkenny Islands Hounds; and the argument that his salary was the equivalent of a carpenter's, at 5 shillings and five pence three farthings a week, made little impression. Discussion ranged over the cost of training a "medical man," the dangers of death from infections, and the frequency with which Boxwell was called from his bed at night. Arthur spoke from experience on the latter and Boxwell got his rise.

In June Arthur sailed away from "board room business," from collections for the Protestant Orphans' Society, from Commons, drunk in the pantry, from the Courts and financial bother, which made it look as though he might have to sell Corsair and the hounds. A warm summer cruise brought relief from the tedium, but also "water closet troubles" in the ladies cabin on Whit Monday.

In early July he was back at the dispensary, where Boxwell was under attack for allowing the nurse-tender to live in without consulting the Guardians. Arthur thought they were motivated by jealousy and was glad to sail away in mid July leaving Frances, pregnant again, in the house at Dunmore which she had taken for three months.

He was not back in Kingstown until October 3rd where he found his wife and children waiting at the train and "all well, thank God."(21) Together they drove home and the year concluded with the simple entry for Christmas Day, "stayed up with Fan in the evening."

The final page contains notes of expenditure for part of the year. "Mrs K's" allowance for January was a £110 and for March £100. His yacht club subscriptions were £2 3s and he spent £2 2s 11d on stamps. There were loans from "Mrs K," one of £11 and one of £7, and subscriptions of £5 each from "Mrs K" and Lady Harriet to the Borris clothing club.

13. THE UNCERTAIN YEARS

The year 1860 began on a very wet Sunday. Arthur
didn't go to church and didn't get up until noon. He
read the papers to Frances, took her out for a drive in
the afternoon and sat with her in the evening. The next
morning was fine and he rode into Bagnelstown before
breakfast. Heavy rains fell again the next day; it was
"pouring." The Dispensary meeting "lasted a long time"
and afterwards Arthur "took a walk round the brook
to look at the floods."(1)

At the end of January their first daughter, Eva Mary,
was christened in the chapel at Borris, and at 1 pm
Frances was "churched." She was soon out riding again
on 'Tinker', and Arthur proudly drove her to inspect
the new cottages he had designed and which were now
completed. His generosity prompted Sir Charles Russel
to describe him several years later to the Parnell
Commission as a "landlord of landlords" who provided
the poor with roomy, comfortable and well slated
accommodation. One of the cottages would have fitted
easily into the drawing room at Borris House, and the
whole row into the Long Gallery of Kilkenny Castle
where Lady Harriet, now released from her duties as
Mistress of Borris, "week ended" with Lady Ormonde,
her great aunt.

Frances encouraged the villagers to plant flowers and
soon, around the doors of Arthur's model cottages, roses
bloomed, making Borris "one of the prettiest villages
in Ireland," or less tactfully put, "like a neat English
village."(2) Inside their new dwellings the women made
lace under Frances' supervision, using patterns brought
from Greece many years earlier by Lady Harriet, and
adapted for the making of Borris Lace. It was intended
that women should supplement the family income by this
new cottage industry, but making lace at the end of the
day, or between caring for families unaided by servants,
seemed to some a further imposition rather than a fresh
opportunity.

The Kavanaghs' list of engagements now varied little from year to year. There was a winter ball at Gowran, "lots of people, hot and squashy, got headache; on the whole spent a pleasant evening,"(4) and although he went to bed at four thirty a.m. he was out early in freezing weather to lay out improvements at Johnson's gate.(3) Gowran was followed by a County Ball for the Protestant Orphan's Society in the Club house in Carlow, under the new 'gasaliers', which were far less attractive than the chandeliers they replaced.

Arthur suffered from chest problems early in 1860 and had to abandon the hunt while Boxwell, who had fallen and sprained his ankle, hobbled about on crutches. Arthur sat with him when he was "seedy" and "had a yarn" with him.(4) By February 10th the doctor was well enough for Arthur to hand over the hunt cards and management of the hunt while he went on a short cruise, taking care that he "gave Fan her jewellery from the safe" before he left.(5)

He was back in Calshott on the 22nd February eagerly receiving a letter from Frances, and on the 26th visited his mother at 21 Suffolk Street, finding her "seedy" and suffering from the effects of opium prescribed by her doctor. He travelled back to Ireland by train from Euston to Holyhead with a rough passage to Kingstown, only to find Frances "seedy" from back pains, and his Aunt Louisa "huffed with me for some reason."(6)

It was a winter of sickness among tenants and Arthur and Frances rode out to visit them. John Doyle was "very sick." Arthur returned to see him bringing with him Boxwell, but found Doyle "very much better." Aunt Louisa brought alarming news of Lady Harriet's health; "very bad account of mother, very ill with erysipelas."(7)

On his birthday there was further catastrophe. "Fan summoned me to her room and told me that the big housemaid had had a child and it was concealed in a box in her room - sent for the doctor who came over and found the brat dead: no marks of violence: woman

confined on Saturday night in the same room as two
older women who were asleep - sent over for the police
sergeant and directed him to go for the coroner; sealed
up the body of the child and afterwards turned in."(8)
The housemaid subsequently appeared in the Magistrates
Court and was committed to the Quarter Sessions on a
charge of concealing the birth of a child. The outcome
is not recorded but the punishment was usually
imprisonment.

Arthur spent Easter in London at 42 Half Moon Street.
He and Hoddy's husband were preparing for a cruise and
Lady Harriet, staying at the Queens Hotel in Norwood,
was still far from well. Palm Sunday was bright and
blowy and while the Trenches went to church, Arthur
read to his mother and sister. The day following he took
the Trench girls, one of whom was Sarah, his biographer,
to the Crystal Palace to hear Piccolomini. He enjoyed it
but found the rest of the concert "stupid." There were
several visits to the Crystal Palace that week, and he
coaxed Lady Harriet to go with him. He records here a
painful incident: "Saw Madame Khore in the crowd but
she ran away the moment she saw us." Despite his good
looks, wit and charm there were those who were repelled
or fascinated by him. He was suffering from toothache
regularly at this time and seemed generally less able to
tolerate daily irritations. A Mr Wynn annoyed him by
staring at him in church. "Mr Wynn stared as bad as
ever," he wrote, and he dismissed Mr MacDonald, the
preacher, as a "stupid conceited man."(9)

He travelled back to Ireland on the crowded Holyhead
train and equally crowded boat, and spent the night
wrapped in his cloak, seated on the hot plate next to
the funnel, a "snug spot."(10) Before leaving Dublin he
visited the Custom House vaults to buy cases of sherry.

One of his distractions during 1860 was photography.
He bought the latest equipment at Knights in Foster
Lane near St Pauls, but achieved only moderate success
in his efforts to take pictures. Lizzie Newton, the wife
of a local magistrate, proved to be the least photogenic

of his subjects. "Two attempts at Lizzie Newton, both failures. After tiffin made two more attempts."(11) A week later there were two more attempts at Lizzie Newton both equally in vain; on 27th April "successful picture of Dick and a faint one of Crystal Pakenham; after tiffin Lizzie Newton - in vain - toothache." His picture of Boxwell on his horse was only "tolerable" and he noted, perhaps with some relief, that the photographer who came over to take pictures of the house "failed owing to bad light."(12)

In 1860 he sold his yacht Corsair and replaced it by R.Y.S. Eva, a schooner of 130 tons built for him by Inmans of Lymington. Like his mother on the Nile, he referred to her as his "wooden home."(13) Corsair had brought him into conflict with the customs officers, whom he saw as a "disagreeable race."(14) They had charged him with smuggling and sailing under a false name. Sailing for Norway with bonded stores, he had been forced by bad weather to return to Kingstown, where the vessel had been searched by a customs officer. "I had nothing save that he expected a tip which I refused to give." Arthur returned home by train and Corsair and her crew sailed for Ross. The bonded stores were forfeited for improper use, but when it was found that only the tobacco had been opened, Arthur received an apology. The charge of sailing under a false name was pursued.

The vessel had been registered as the Triumvir, and to give any other name than that on her certificate of registration was illegal. Arthur, meticulous as ever, although renaming the ship Corsair and decorating the crew's head-bands with that name, when asked officially at every port of call, had given the name Triumvir. He was gleeful at his defeat of officialdom, but attributed the incident as much to his own "high minded stinginess as anything else."(15)

The winter of 1860 was a bad one. There were thick fogs, 17 degrees of frost and fuel was short. While the tenants froze, Arthur sailed on December 1st on his new yacht Eva for the warmer waters of the Mediterranean. Frances and the boys took the steamer to Malta and joined him there, to spend Christmas Day sheltering in their cabins from the rains and squalls before sailing on to Corfu.

The Kavanagh s remained in the Mediterranean through the spring and well into summer. Arthur loved Albania, and he wrote, "Its very beauty was a drawback to the sportsman, with the lovely Mediterranean heath eight to ten feet high covered with its white snow-bells - the rhododendrons, caurustinus, arlutus vying with each other in the richness of their blossoms; the Judas tree with its bright scarlet twigs and leaves . . . "(16)

"He was," writes Frances, "quite dependant upon the miserable horses of that country to carry him about, as no English horse could with safety have got over the hill-tracks, which were very steep and often slippery.

"At Avalona only one horse could be procured for him - and that a mere bag of bones. Starting on this wretched beast to a covert where a pig was reported to be, he was accompanied by the Greek beater and the sailors, while I walked close behind him. It was most unusual for him to ride near the rest of the party, for generally he preferred to keep quite away from them, as by doing so he had a better chance of shots. We had not gone far up a steep mountain-path, where every now and then the horse, ever responsive to his call, had to spring up rocky steps fit only for goats, when just as we reached a spot with a precipice at one side many hundreds of feet down to the sea, the horse attempted one of these jumps, failed, and rolled over the brink. A small cactus bush about ten feet below checked Arthur's fall, and Arthur quite calmly called to the sailors to unstrap him from the saddle. This they did, being able to climb down where few others could have ventured, and hoisted him up to the path, while the poor horse rolled down and was instantaneously killed.

"This did not shake Arthur's nerve in the least, for next

day he rode over a still more impracticable mountain, and distanced all his party, till at last I overtook him, though in doing so the sharp rocks had cut through the soles of my boots, and I was almost barefoot."(17)

Arthur wrote, "I daresay it would not have been a painful death, but there is something more than usually awful in it that I do not fancy - something peculiarly exciting to the nerves in looking down a dizzy abyss and then finding you are going over it."(18)

On this cruise, on the eve of his thirtieth birthday he wrote, "This is my last of the twenties; to-morrow (D.V.) the thirties begin. What a ten years to review! When I began them, a homeless wanderer in India; what mercies I have had showered upon me! Have I tried to use and not abuse them? Have I cared for the people committed to my charge? Have I tried to make myself useful, and duly to fill the position in which I have been placed? Hard questions to answer. I have tried: but have I looked to God to help me, to give me patience, to encourage me when I have been weary and disgusted, to make me thankful for what I had, and not longing for things I had not?"(19)

In July 1861 Arthur returned to Borris to the "hearty demonstrations" of joy by the tenants; to the customary bonfires, illuminations and "the crowds assembled to cheer him." "Poor people!" he wrote, "they must like me; but how I have deserved that they should do so I cannot think. God grant me grace to cherish their affection and to guard it as a precious blessing one can never prize enough, or guard too jealously."(20)

If the tenantry were resentful of his increasing absences they were not showing it, and almost immediately he returned to the tasks he found wearying. The Summer Assizes, the days of "fiscal business" on the Grand Jury, and sitting in judgement on local villains. One of his own name, Margaret Kavanagh, "found" a neighbour's purse in her basket; another local man was judged guilty of "uttering" base sixpences, while the drunken boatmen on the river Barrow had to be dealt with for theft of freight.

There was light relief in watching Boxwell's cricket eleven, but more tedium in store when he was proposed as chairman of the New Ross Board of Guardians by Mr Sweetman, a Catholic whom Arthur regarded as a "humbug." Arthur had doubts about his acceptability, but after some opposition he was elected. According to Sweetman he was "most painstaking and just, and in his decisions in any case that came before him his religion or politics could not be discovered." He was always anxious that the Catholic chaplain's applications should be attended to and "his action in this matter was much and favourably spoken off."(21) Mass was normally said in the Poor House dining room, a practice deplored by the Catholic guardians. Sweetman proposed the building of a Catholic chapel but the cost estimated at between £300 to £400 was seen as prohibitive. Arthur dismissed the objections saying "If we build anything, let us build something we need not be ashamed of." When the new chapel, the first of its kind since emancipation, was completed, "Mr Kavanagh came up to see it and was greatly pleased," says Sweetman.

14.   ESCAPE TO SEA

In 1862 Arthur was invited to stand as a Parliamentary candidate. He was dissatisfied with the "parochialism" of his role as Master of Borris, and believed he could contribute to and influence the interminable debates about Ireland and the land problems at a national level. Frances, who now showed her steely nature, opposed the idea. " . . . I have to acknowledge that I used all my influence to keep him back. It seemed to me that, accustomed as he was to a life of constant exercise in the open air, the confinement of Parliament would be most injurious to him."(1) Arthur gave way and turned to the sea for consolation.

He set out for Corfu in October 1862. The 29th of the month "dawned upon the slumbering mortals with a day break as watery looking as one could wish to see excepting that it was not raining; a circumstance which is supposed to be rather worthy of note in Ireland." For several days he was marooned aboard his "wooden home" watching the "dissipated old sun" lighting up the ruins of Dunbrody Abbey and attempting to tinge with gold "the tapering masts, gossamer-like rigging, long low hull of a schooner yacht as she lay at anchor in the Waterford river, waiting for a wind that was "not a regular gale in our teeth."(2)

Once underway Arthur felt free. "There is," he wrote, " . . . no more exhilarating sense, no more thorough realisation of the word of freedom than to be skimming over the boundless ocean - the trackless deep with a good ship under one, free to go where one likes, the boundary of the great sea ones only limit."(3)

He was happy to shake off the chores of a landlord and the tensions of living in a divided society. "No more post bags full of stupid wearisome letters that must be answered. No more Poor Law meetings ugh! How I hate them with their bickerings and jealousies, and worse

than all, the curse of this wretched country - Bigotry
displaying itself at every turn and from every side;
everyone convinced that everyone else wants to convert
the whole community to his plan of going to heaven, or
elsewhere." Sessions, assizes, elections, railway boards;
the list is endless, with their inseparable train of worries
and annoyances all left behind on the "dull unchanging
shore."(4)

On board the Eva, named after his elder daughter,
he was free to enjoy the company of his crew sitting
out on dry nights watching the clouds of "baccy smoke"
ascending or being blown away leeward. He relished the
company of an unnamed friend with whom he eventually
travelled thousands of miles, and the company of the
skipper who "was as good a sailor as ever walked a
deck or whistled to a salty wind;" and old Neddy the
cook, who was so tall that when Arthur first saw him
emerging from the forehatch, he wondered how much
more of him was to come. Tradition had it that when
Neddy fell overboard in the Bay of Biscay he touched
bottom and was not drowned. Always with them were
the dogs: Vido a terrier trained to hunt pigs, the terror
of many an unfortunate "porker," and Trap surnamed
Jeremiah because of his "lacrimose cast of countenance."

Renewing his acquaintance with Gibraltar, Johnny
Spaniard and the Rock scorpions, his ears "addled" by
a babble of foreign tongues, he "jumped" into a gig,
stopping only at Black Charley's to spend loose change
on trinkets, before driving to the Alameda to see the
"beau monde." Here he paused to listen to the band
and watched the Spanish beauties, whose eyes he likened
to those of a gazelle and hair to a raven's wing, "and
indulge ad libitum in such like trash. But in all sincerity,
I have no admiration for their foreign graces; our English
girls alone possess that style of beauty which can ever
squeeze a drop of sentimentality out of my briney old
heart. Whatever quarter of the globe I may be in, I
love to look upon a real English lady; her beauty may
not be brilliant, but the charm of a gentle and refined
mind places her beyond comparison."(5)

At about the same time, making notes for his book on his cruises, Arthur wrote in respect of the new Iron ships, " . . . it is for me and every other Englishman to hope that those new Iron ships will keep as long unsullied and untarnished that British Flag which (as the song says)" has for a thousand years on our old wooden walls braved victorious "the battle and the breeze." In these generalisations Arthur betrays how far he had moved from his Irishness to identify with the "foreign occupier."

Describing a race with another schooner, which he refers to as G, he shows his zest for a contest. In a mixture of metaphors he describes RYS Eva merrily skimming like a bird over the huge waves and "flying through the water like a racehorse, stern sinking into the deep leaden-coloured valleys." She showed "her wild joy by her mad race through a sheet of creaming seething foam." It was a pretty sight for it was a fair sea-going race; none of your large jibs; none of your top sails; but blowing a gale of wind, the whole sea covered with ragged streaky foam, the beautiful range of the Sierra Nevada with its snow capped ridge gilded by the rays of the now setting sun; and these two frail looking vessels, defying the rage of the elements to entice each other." He records with glee that "as eight bells went, we showed our light, and had the satisfaction of being answered by our adversary - well astern!"(6)

Off Palermo Arthur mused on the early annexation of the two Sicilies by Italy. Every man, woman and child, he thought, believed the millenium had dawned and that they would be rich without exertion. Like the rebels in Marseilles in 1848, they had come to acknowledge this was not so and he concluded with the predictable comment of a rich Irish landlord that there are no riches without individual exertion.

At Naples Frances and the children came on board having travelled overland and they spent Christmas together. Walter was now almost seven. The early pessimistic diagnoses about his health seemed to be proving unfounded. Young Arthur was five and Eva two. For Christmas Day their cabins were decorated with ilex, orange, and myrtle, and they all wore their best clothes and ate roast beef and plum pudding.

Once in Ionian waters the enthusiastic sailor became an enthusiastic sportsman, with his usual keenness for game and particularly "porkers." He loved the Albanian sheep dogs, "very powerful, savage, half wild, they are the most formidable assailant; indeed their attack is the greatest danger one has to encounter in Albanian shooting; even in self defence you dare not kill them as their lives are rated far above a man's."(7) He tells how fifteen guard dogs stationed themselves around two hundred sheep and no animal or man dared approach them. He recalled one of them in particular:

"I remember watching one hoary patriarch sitting at his post . . . he seemed . . . as if his mind had wandered back to the adventures and scenes of his past life . . . He was disturbed from his reverie by a little lamb staggering up to him and falling against his shaggy side. He turned his great head round and looked at the little beast licking his old chops as much as to say, 'I should like awfully to eat you but am in honour bound to defend you;' and to avoid temptation he got up and stalked away."(8)

A demonstration on one of the islands in favour of Union with Greece, irritated Arthur and brought out his dislike of agitators, particularly foreign ones. "It was," he wrote sarcastically, "one of those smothered throes of agony felt by a free spirit groaning under a tyrant's yoke." Such manifestations he believed, if successful in drawing large crowds, usually led to bloodshed; and if unsuccessful, were an opportunity for pick pockets. He gently mocked the black-eyed, black-moustachioed men in narrow brimmed hats, "Noah's Ark" coats buttoned across the chest and "peg top" trousers. Their ties were indescribable and they had the air of the cast of a comic opera. Like all the southern races they seemed prone to take offence, to be "over huffy" and "peppery," and the outcome of their irritable excitable and narrow "little minds" was behaviour excusable only in a "spoilt or sickly child." Arthur didn't like them and he didn't like their cause, and with a dash of snobbery consoled himself that the true owners of the soil, the landed gentry, did not welcome these moves towards Greece.(9)

Frances and the boys enjoyed these trips as much as Arthur. "We all liked the climate of Corfu, and the sport on the opposite shore of Albania afforded Arthur the keenest pleasure, in which we all participated, accompanying him as far as possible, and when tired, either resting on the ground or climbing into one of the splendid ilex trees with which that country abounds, where, out of sight and scent of the game, we often saw far more than the sportsmen. The interest of watching wild animals when they fancied themselves unobserved was unfailing, and the return in the evening to the yacht was always pleasant. An excellent well-cooked dinner awaited us, and then music (which Arthur always passionately loved) closed the day."(10)

They enjoyed themselves coaxing Albanian women to pose, and Arthur created panic among a group of them when he showed them their sisters upside down in the lens. They ran away shrieking and holding down their skirts for they thought they had posed "upside down."

Adventures were numerous; "the ladies" enjoyed seeing Turks in a "state of nature," not naked Arthur hastened to add, but in their natural habitat. The men enjoyed bathing in canvas tubs on deck which Arthur found refreshing and invigorating, if not comfortable; dried by a keen wind they went to breakfast very hungry.

Sadly their pet monkey ate arsenic paste off grape skins which they were preserving. Against Arthur's inclinations a local doctor put the animal in a bag and dosed it with castor oil. The monkey did not survive and was buried at sea with full naval honours, though deprived of a salvo of artillery because of passing ships.

Frances returned to Borris overland, and Arthur sailed for New Ross arriving in March 1863. Frances drove to meet him and leaves this account: "As the car on which he was drew near, I saw that on the driver's seat sat a very large ape, which filled me with dismay. Savage to all others, he was quite gentle with Arthur, and perfectly devoted to him. On one occasion he broke his chain and made his way to the nursery - nurses and children flying before him in terror. The 'Master' was sent for to dislodge him but, on arriving, it was many minutes before he could speak for laughing. There on the middle of the table sat Jack, one paw deep in a cream-jug, looking blissfully content. However, at one word from his master, he quietly returned to his own quarters, to every one's relief. There he often received visits from strangers, who sometimes found to their cost that Jack was not to be treated with too great familiarity."

"One lady, heedless of warning, ventured to approach him, when Jack put out his paw and seized a string of pearls she wore round her neck and put them into his mouth; and great was the trouble his master had to make him disgorge them."(11)

Jack was a favourite with Arthur and like the brown bear given him as a cub, sat with him under an Oak in the Courtyard when he "held court," reading letters for the villagers, sometimes helping to write them, hearing their confessions, soothing troubled minds and acting as intermediary. In this Courtyard, to Arthur's grief, Jack died tragically. A house party was leaving for a day's shooting in the demesne. Among them was an Italian, resident in Ireland. "Out into the yard," writes Sarah Steele, "stepped il bravo cacciatore," ready for "le sport," which he facetiously commenced by levelling his gun. The gun went off accidentally blowing off Jack's head and just missing a groom. "I do not think, however," says Mrs Steele, of the Italian "he was ever invited to join another shooting party there."(12)

Bessy, the brown bear, another of Arthur's pets,

eventually grew too big to be handled at Borris, and Arthur gave her to the 1st Life Guards who, not entirely appreciative, sent her back. Arthur then reluctantly gave her to Dublin Zoo.

Busier each year with local duties, and devoting more and more time to fishing, sometimes in the brook but also in the Westmeath Lakes and Lough Arrow in Sligo, and more and more time to sailing, Arthur sold his hunters and his pack of harriers.

The summer of 1864 was spent sailing in the Arctic. He wrote daily to Frances describing events. "On the 7th my watch was the morning one - flat calm. V was on deck with me, and we were trying to fish in two hundred and eighty fathoms of water (at least that is the depth that the chart gives), when we spied two white things skimming along under the bottom of the ship. I thought they were two skates or flat fish, but they turned out to be the two fins of a whale. He passed under us and, giving himself a tumble on the other side of the vessel, soon showed what he was. He gave another swim around us, coming then close alongside, so near that he could be touched with a boathook. He gradually let his tail sink down till he was in a perpendicular posture, with his head over the water. There he remained for nearly five minutes having a quiet look at us. It was flat calm, and the water quite clear, so that we could see his whole form quite distinctly - about twenty five feet long, and big in proportion. I don't think he was a regular whale, but more of the black fish species. Certainly, if any one else had described such a scene to me, I should not have believed him."(13)

He was moved by the sight of a little girl rowing. "One party we met coming in from a bank about fourteen miles out to sea, where he had been fishing all day with only a little girl about eight years old in the boat with him. She was pulling the two stroke oars (skulls) by which these boats are steered, and splendidly she did it, pulling as long and steady a stroke as her father.

Poor little child! We gave her a lot of sugar and sweet biscuits, at which she was greatly pleased, and insisted on shaking hands with H, who gave them to her."(14)

The scenery was "very grand" - "black scraggy mountains with sharp peaks of every conceivable shape and form rising from one to three thousand feet out of the fiord, which is about a mile wide. All the valleys and crevices are filled with snow, which has hardly begun to melt at all yet."

"The sky is all clouded and wild-looking, which keeps up the sombre character of the scene, and the wind off the snow makes one's teeth chatter."

"Suddenly the fiord takes a turn, so that the sides of the hills are exposed to the sun, and the whole scene is changed as if by magic - hardly a vestige of snow to be seen. The hills sloping up from the water are clothed with the bright green of the young birch - first-rate looking covert! A cascade here and there drains off the water from the snow that is melting. On the top of the hill a settlement of wooden houses, a church, and the parson's house complete the contrast." (15)

On the longest day they entered the Arctic Circle, and on 6th July began their fishing at a settlement near the mouth of the Pavrig river. "The mosquitos were dreadful," and Arthur was unlucky and "killed nothing." One of his companions, known as H, killed four salmon, one over forty lbs, the other over twenty. Arthur fished from a small boat, the others from the shore. There was little prospect of shooting for "white grouse and black game exist but in no very great number . . . " "Seals are almost a myth. On the whole journey we have only seen four or five."(16) Arthur's luck changed on the 17th July and he had the best days fishing I ever had, or, I suppose ever will have. I killed eight salmon weighing one hundred and sixty six lbs to my own rod." H had killed the largest and Arthur came second with a "thirty six pounder." Arthur was responsible for feeding the crew with his catch, as the others had to give theirs to a local headman; he stored dried fish for the voyage, finding it impossible to get meat in Russian Lapland.

The sight of the child in the boat in the Arctic seems to have touched a gentle chord in Arthur. A third son, Charles, had been born just before his departure and the other children, Walter, Eva and Mary were growing up aware that their father while different, could do all the things that other fathers did. Arthur wrote to Walter from the Arctic encouraging him to be good and asking "Have you caught any shrimps yet? How are Arthur, Eva and Mary and Master Charlie? I suppose he is not able to speak yet. Give them all my fondest love."(16) Even with the joy of his growing family, the satisfaction of public office in his county and his many pleasures, Arthur remained unfulfilled.

15. PARLIAMENT

Palmerston died in 1865 and was succeeded by Lord
Russel as Prime Minister, with Gladstone as leader of
the House of Commons. The transition to democracy
had begun but not without faltering. Gladstone's bid for
Parliamentary reform failed, and the Government were
driven from office. Extending the franchise and enabling
electors to vote in secret, accountable no longer to the
landlord, were again key issues, particularly in Ireland,
where eviction was an easy option for a displeased
landlord.

The Anglican Church, established by law as the Church
of Ireland, was generously endowed. It was seen by
Catholics as a church of conquest and was associated
by both Catholics and Presbyterians with a "territorial
aristocracy." Supported financially by Catholics and
Presbyterians through compulsory tithes, it was a very
vulnerable institution. Change was in the air for the
privileged Church of the minority.

Land, not religion, was the burning question for the
Irish at this time. The Carlow Post took the view that
"if the Irish Church was disestablished tomorrow there
would be as much and as little of the Royal Supremacy
in Ireland as before. In England, improvements to a
holding were generally carried out by the landlord; in
Ireland improvements were generally carried out by the
tenant, who had no security of tenure and could readily
be evicted without compensation for his improvements.
Since the Famine, recognizing the greater efficiency
of larger holdings, some landlords evicted tenants and
combined their farms into more profitable units. The
dispersed tenants drifted into the towns to become a
burden on the rate payers, and as the Irish paid the
Poor Law Rate according to electoral divisions, not
according to a union of divisions, the towns people
considered themselves to be paying dearly for the sins
of their rural counterparts.

The unresolved land question fed "agrarian crime." The agents of unpopular landlords, along with their bailiffs, game keepers and labourers, were sometimes brutally murdered or maimed. James Stephens, one of Smith O'Brien's lieutenants in the '48 rising, claimed in 1865 that 85,000 men were drilling in preparation for revolt As in 1798, Borris House was stocked with food and fortified against attack. As in '48, Arthur rode out at night looking for rebels, while the scurrilous gossiped about a resumption of amorous affairs. He went on fine moonlit nights "over the stone walls, down the mountain-side making the stones fly at every stride, across the brook and through the swamp till he had fairly baffled all pursuit and could sit still and laugh at his ease."(1)

With momentous issues to be decided it was unlikely that Arthur, with his concern for "the soil," his sense of his role among his own people and his natural desire to preserve his own interests, would remain on the side-lines. In Wexford the sitting member of Parliament, Mr George QC was appointed to the Queen's Bench, and if Mr Sweetman's account is to be relied upon, it was in the Poor House at New Ross that the Guardians began discussing a successor. They dismissed their chairman, Arthur Kavanagh, as unwilling to stand; but Sweetman assured them that if pressed by a sufficiently weighty deputation, he would agree. This time Frances raised no objection, and even reproached herself for opposing his parliamentary ambitions in 1862. Arthur did agree, and defeated the "clever and loquacious" John Pope-Hennesy by 2,641 votes to 1,812.(2)

Parliament was opened by Queen Victoria on the 5th February 1867. It was a dismal day, and although she drove in a closed carriage, she was well received by the crowd. On the following day Arthur was sworn and took his seat as member for Wexford County.

"His appearance in the House excited a good deal of curiosity for a time; but he was only a nine day wonder," wrote the Carlow Post. "He now comes and goes without

observation. Yes, but how does he come and go, our
readers may ask. He uses a wheel chair - not through
the lobby to be stared at by strangers, but by a private
door behind the Speakers chair. His servant wheels him
into the division lobby, and arriving at the door leading
into the House on the left of the Speaker, he springs
upon the back of the servant, who drops his burden
upon a seat, by courtesy reserved close to the door."(3)

Later in his Parliamentary career Arthur re-asserted the
right of members to moor their vessels near the Palace
of Westminster, and he was rowed from the RYS Eva to
Speakers steps to enter the palace there. Inside there
was an unspoken agreement that he would not be helped.
With a device fitted to his chair, he made his way along
the corridors and manoeuvred himself around the Commons
library where he wrote his letters "simply and legibly."
"He performs this feat in a curious manner; he puts into
his mouth the top end of the pen, presses it lower down
with his stumps with which he guides it and makes it
fly across the paper with surprising swiftness." (4)

In Arthur's first year as an MP, the Fenian rebels
having failed to provoke a rising in Ireland, brought the
struggle for Ireland's liberty to England. The attempt
to seize Chester Castle failed; a police sergeant was
shot in Manchester during the rescue of Fenian prisoners
from a police van, and a bomb was placed against the
wall of Clerkenwell prison, killing innocent residents in
nearby houses. Arthur took no part in Parliamentary
proceedings at this time, beyond putting down a question
on the lighting of the coast between Carnsore Point
and Wicklow Head and voting against the democratising
clauses of the Representation of the People Bill and the
Established Church (Ireland) Bill. In July 1868 Parliament
was prorogued, and in October the general election
campaign was opened with Disraeli's plea for the return
of the Conservatives to prevent the Pope becoming
master of England. A more rational Gladstone, who
proposed conciliation with Ireland, administrative reform
and disestablishment of the Anglican Church in Ireland,
was returned with a majority of 100 seats.

While Pack-Beresford was in trouble with his electors
for entering his horse, the Fenian, in the Patriotic
Stakes, Arthur, returned unopposed in Carlow, spent
Christmas at Borris. The family was expanding. Having
survived his childhood illnesses, Walter was now twelve
and at Eton; Arthur was eleven, and Eva nine. The
younger girls Mary and Agnes were about to be joined
by another sister, for Frances was once more pregnant.
With her mother-in-law, Lady Harriet, and Lady Harriet's
sister Louisa, she gave a party for children attending
schools on the estate. In the servants' hall, helped by
the family, she dressed an enormous Christmas tree
and at 6 pm "the ladies" met the local children at the
entrance to Borris House. Frances gave out "valuable
premiums to pupils, for regular attendance and needle
work etc," and the children dutifully cheered. Each
child then received a ticket with a number correspond-
ing to the number on "some valuable article on the
tree." Led by Frances, Lady Harriet and Lady Louisa,
they next went to the servants hall where the tree
stood. "Their astonishment and rejoicing on beholding
such a dazzling and to them most unusual sight was
indeed very great."(5) After Frances had given each
child a gift they all sat down to eat cake and fruit.

Arthur made his maiden speech on April 7th 1869
during the Poor Law (Ireland) Amendment Bill, which
sought to extend Union rating to Ireland thus sharing
the burden of supporting the poor between groupings of
electoral divisions, between town and country. The
Commons had listened patiently to the "familiar and
combative utterances of a few Irish members. When a
dozen others started to their legs, the Speaker nodded
in the direction of the opposition benches and said,
"Mr Kavanagh." The effect of the words was, according
to the Liverpool Daily Post, "electrifying" and "every
eye" in the House was turned to the row almost under
the gallery where Arthur sat with his notes resting on
his top hat.

He argued that support for the poor through Union rating
was part of the larger question of general taxation. He

dismissed attempts to draw analogies with Union rating in England, reminding the Government of their assertions during the Irish Church Bill and discussions on the Land Question that, "no analogy existed between the two countries." He believed that it was dire necessity not landlords which drove the poor into the towns. "They fled from their dwellings where pestilence was rife, and starvation stared them in the face, into towns where food was to be had." He also believed that, during the starvation following the potato crop failure, it was poor distribution of food not lack of money that was the problem; now landlords were building to encourage labourers to return to the land, so serious was "the want of labour."(6)

Towns, he said, owed much of their prosperity to the rural districts for which they were a market; he believed the higher value of property more than compensated for the higher rating. He gave comparative figures based on the Ordinance value per acre and rent charged, and concluded that "town man" was richer by £3.3s.6d each year than "rural man." Both Gladstone and the Speaker A J Denison "paid great attention;" and when Arthur flicked over the top sheet of his notes and went on to the next, the House cheered.

"Was the town, then, only to enjoy the advantages of its position?" he asked, and not be responsible for the drawbacks of its mixed population?" Absentee landlords who did nothing to provide work for the poor would be as well off as the landlord who in a neighbouring division "looked after his people, built them houses and perhaps often pinched himself to keep them in employment and keep them off the rates." He concluded by saying that when taxation ceased to be local, a feeling of mistaken charity or a desire to obtain popularity might influence a Guardian in obtaining relief for those very little worse off than those who paid rates. "What was everybody's business was nobody's business."(7)

When he sat down the House cheered. Chichester Fortescue, Chief Secretary for Ireland, acknowledged the Honourable Member for Carlow's knowledge of the question and "power of dealing with it," but did not accept that the measure could be deferred until general taxation was discussed. He did, however, accept that the circumstances of Ireland differed from those of England, and proposed that the Bill be referred to a Select Committee.

The Speaker sent Arthur a note saying, "I offer you my compliments on the excellent manner and tone of your speech, which as you will see has made a very favourable impression on the House."(8) The Liverpool Daily Post added, "Judging by the matter of his first address and the manner in which it was received it may reasonably be predicted that Mr Kavanagh, who belongs constitutionally to that type of men which wins in public life, the men with large heads and deep chests and faces full of force, will often be heard with advantage in the House of Commons."(9)

Arthur was heard frequently on the subject of Union rating throughout his Parliamentary career. The matter was before the House again in 1873, but with few new arguments on either side except Arthur's. He alleged that the report before the House was at variance with the evidence, for the committee preparing it had failed to find an appropriate chairman and had instead elected one who favoured change, thus putting those opposed to Union rating in a permanent minority. Arthur found himself attacked for treating the matter as one of money, when in reality it was a matter of justice. Representatives of Irish trade pointed out that while every struggling tradesman paid income-tax, tenants of the landed gentry did not, though many were rich. The Government, it was alleged, was afraid of the "landed interest, and there the matter rested for the time being."(10)

The issue came up again in the next Parliament, and Arthur was less gently treated than at the time of his maiden speech. In the debate on the Poor Relief (Ireland) Bill he was shouted down when he said, with little supporting evidence, that the people of Ireland were opposed to change. Mr Dunbar, Member for New Ross, acknowledged that Arthur was Chairman of the Poor Law Guardians, but he, Mr Dunbar, would represent the views of the townspeople. He was not surprised that Mr Kavanagh opposed the Bill; there was no gentleman in Ireland with more reasons to be thankful for the present state of the law. The rates on Mr Kavanagh's property had been reduced from 4s 2d to 8d. Mr Dunbar went on to list division after division in which rates in the areas where Arthur Kavanagh held property had been reduced, and he attributed this to the "clearing" of estates between 1854 and 1873; the period of Arthur's tenure at Borris. While it was true that as a land owner Arthur benefited from the present law it was inaccurate to say that he had driven labourers from his estates into the towns. In an earlier debate, he had challenged Mr Dunbar's predecessor to give an instance of clearance on the Borris estates and he had failed to do so.

Gladstone introduced his Land Bill in 1870 aiming to end some of the injustices peculiar to Ireland by providing for tenants to be compensated for improvements they had made to their holdings and for their protection against capricious eviction. Arthur took a line independent of his own Conservative party giving cautious support to the Government's main proposals. He clashed with Disraeli who sought to limit the Bill's provisions but complained that his "consistency" was put to the test by the Government's compensation provision for improvements which he saw as too high especially for richer tenant farmers. He felt most strongly on the question of subletting and moved an amendment to the Bill to outlaw it. Sub-letting, he told the House, led to "middlemen" charging exorbitant rents for miserable hovels with floors inches deep in mud, without windows or chimneys, with walls propped up with sticks and roofs "only sufficient to keep out the sun." In his seventeen years as a landlord, ten of which were spent acting as his own agent, the most frequent disputes he had had to deal with were between middlemen and their labourers. The farmer generally alleged idleness on the part of the labourer whom he asked to evict, the latter alleged meanness on the part of the middleman; too mean, said Arthur, to provide "a wisp of straw to repair a roof."(11) His own labourers were in the main his direct tenants; a situation he had brought about gradually as leases fell vacant. He had built eighty six new cottages, carried out repairs and improved sanitation at a cost of £400. His neighbours Captain Beresford and Colonel Tighe and his honourable colleague Lord Bessborough were all doing the same, but tenants with a small acreage usually lacked the finance to build adequate dwellings for their employees. For that reason he opposed sub-letting and hoped that minimum standards for labourers would be laid down.

The suave Chichester-Fortescue, in replying, said that the Government was sorry that it found itself in opposition to the honourable member for Carlow, but he hoped he would not insist on a measure that might inflict a penalty on a farmer if his cottage had an insufficient chimney or a window that did not open. Arthur took the point. He had given the house a good hearted, emotive, even defensive account of his steward-ship, arguing as though his own particular experience was general to the landlord class. He cared for his work-force and being astute like his grandfather Lord Clancarty, realised that happy and comfortable tenants were an asset to the estate, however many of his contemporaries showed no such insight.

There was a humorous interlude in the debate when he noticed an omission, through a misprint in the text of the Bill, which he said would entitle tenants to claim compensation on improvements on reclamation since the time of the Flood. Chistester Fortescue assured him that the appropriate amendment would be made.

In May 1870 a mob, or an orderly meeting, according the point of view, gathered in the forecourt of the Catholic chapel just down hill from the main gate of Borris House, and listened to Father Carey, the parish priest, speak on the "Borris evictions." Mr Little, a tenant of Lord Castlecomer, had evicted an eighty

year old blind man named Byrne. The nationalist press
reminded its readers that "poor old Byrne" came from
a family as ancient as the Kavanaghs and the O'Tooles,
and that "persecuting and exterminating" landlords had
sent more persons to their premature graves in a few
years than "agrarian assassins" would in a hundred. Byrne,
who had farmed his lands for a lifetime, was no longer
fit for work. He had paid his rent but had received,
along with his rent receipts, notice of eviction; he had
accommodated his landlord in the past by giving up a
proportion of his land to enable the river bank to be
straightened. When Mr Little alleged that Byrne had
not cared for his sheep properly, the "Wexford People"
replied that if he required a shepherd, he should employ
one. Little defended himself saying he had a "right to
do as he liked with his labourers if they did not do his
business," and that he had provided more work in the
area than many, with the exception of Arthur Kavanagh.
Byrne countered that the complainants were acting in
anticipation of the new land legislation, trying to evict
him while they could. Father Carey felt it necessary
to tell strangers present that this meeting was called at
Borris simply for convenience, and "has nothing to say
to Mr Kavanagh, the worthy landlord of the soil, for he
is considered a fair landlord and puts out no one who
pays his rent and in some cases makes allowance for
improvements and compensates his tenantry." Arthur was
already putting into practice the provisions of the Land
Bill and the priests remarks brought cheers. "But", he
went on, "the best trait of his character is that he is
kind to the poor, and may the prayers of the poor be
heard for his welfare."(12)

When further land legislation was introduced in 1876
Arthur opposed it as a Fenian plot, designed to deprive
landlords of estates they held, not through forfeiture,
but from time immemorial. It was an ill-informed view,
for most Irish landlords held their lands as a result of
dispossession of others for political or religious reasons.
While the Kavanaghs had held extensive lands from "time
immemorial" Borris itself had been forfeited by the Ryans
in the Kavanaghs' favour.

Arthur told the House of Commons during the debate on the Land Tenure Bill that he now regretted his support for the 1870 Land Act. He believed it treated Irish tenants as imbeciles in need of the protection of law in negotiations of rents, when the bonds forged with landlords over generations were more effective. "In days gone by their forefathers went to mine for help in trouble, for advice in difficulty, sure of a willing hand and a sympathetic ear; and now their children came to me."(13) It was a partial view based on sentimental recollections of the tenant gatherings of his youth and his own comfortable relationship with his tenants.

As each year passed, Arthur became increasingly alarmed at the land reform proposals seeing them as "communistic" and a capitulation to agitation which was Ireland's downfall, and which had stained her soil with blood and made her a byword among nations.(14)

16.   AGITATION AND ADULATION

Land legislation did little to calm agitation in Ireland, and consequently Law and Order or "Peace Preservation" became an increasingly important issue. Arthur saw agitation and the weak governmental response to it as twin evils. A prisoner of his class he could not concede that perhaps the "agitators" had a point of view, and were articulating the legitimate grievances of others. On St Patrick's Day 1869 he drew the attention of the Chief Secretary for Ireland to a leading article in 'The People', a Wexford paper, which he read to the House. "If a few landlords have been shot or shot at, perhaps by men maddened by their inhumanity" this is "nothing compared with the dreadful murders constantly committed in England; we are told forsooth that this constitutes a 'reign of terror,' and legislation of a severely coercive nature is just now the one thing needful for Ireland. But these sanguinary champions of the 'right of property,' as they call them, as if Providence ever endowed one man, or one set of men with 'the right' to defraud another, seem to forget, that according to the whole civilised world, evicting landlords deserved to be hanged not shot." 'The People' went on to deplore assassination, even of one of these "territorial ogres, whose ruthless cruelty seems to exclude them from the pale of civil society," and asked, "if the terror does reign who are to blame?" The people of Ireland were absolved and the landlords, "the men who have shown no mercy to the people," condemned.(1)

An indignant Arthur asked the First Secretary if he considered that words such as these, directly inciting to violence, should be used with impunity. Chichester Fortescue's reply was brief. He did not think such words should be used with impunity, but refused to be drawn into commenting on an "isolated passage."

A year later Chichester-Fortescue introduced his own Peace Preservation Bill, and found an impassioned

supporter in the honourable member for Carlow. Some
Peace Preservation legislation involving suspension of
Habeus Corpus and the arbitrary arrest of suspects had
previously been passed in 1866; now further legislation
was proposed. Arthur came to this debate furnished
with letters from a Mr Nicholas of County Meath, who
could not get fire insurance, so great were the risks to
property; and with quotations from the Reverend Thomas
Doyle, a speaker at an Enniscorthy tenants' rights
meeting, presided over by Lord Grannard. Father Doyle
preached agrarian heresy and Arthur unwittingly gave
him a platform in the Imperial Parliament. The "great
God alone had absolute ownership of the soil," said
Doyle. "Was earth created for kings, emperors or for
governments? No, No. Was it created for an aristocracy
or an oligarchy of buckeens?" The land on the contrary,
he argued, was made for the people who were released
from their allegiance when governments abused their
trust by putting land out to oligarchies. Father Doyle
foolishly concluded by quoting John Mitchel, "If the
landlord evict you, shoot him like a mad dog," and
"if the landlord hides in London, shoot the agent."(2)

Arthur was enraged at what he saw as a lack of
even-handedness in the treatment of agitators. Orange
processions, he said, were banned and their leaders
imprisoned; and while he denied an 'Orange' connection,
deploring all provocative acts, he believed that if the
Earl of Grannard had been an Orangeman and Father
Doyle a clergyman of the disestablished Church, they
would have been apprehended and punished.

Gladstone, calm among the heated debaters, pointed out
that the Peace Preservation Bill was not a measure to
protect landlords, since the vast majority of the victims
of The Land War were labourers, stewards and keepers.
Four hundred and twenty five members voted for the
Bill, and only thirteen against.

Arthur's intervention in yet another "Peace Preservation"
debate in 1875 showed how out of touch he was with the
feelings of the Irish people. They were grateful, he told

the House, for "the charity and generosity" with which England went to the aid of Ireland in the Famine years. Without this aid they would not have lived to rebel, but died of want. Fenianism had disappeared in Carlow under coercive legislation; coercive only to those who sought to murder or administer unlawful oaths, or write unlawful letters. His "florid references" were increasingly seen as irrelevant to the debates, but he was acknowledged as one of a race of kind and beneficent landlords who allowed their tenants to live and prosper but who were untypical of their class.(3)

In June 1876 Mr Isaac Butt, leader of the Home Rule party, moved that "a Select Committee be appointed to inquire and report on the nature, the extent, and the grounds of the demand made by a large proportion of the Irish people for the restoration to Ireland of an Irish Parliament, with power to control the internal affairs of that country."(4)

In this debate an increasingly angry Arthur imputed bad faith to the Home Rulers, accusing them of introducing the subject simply to ferment agitation. He rejected the notion of the "Divine Right" of every nation to govern itself, and postulated that God would not have given such a right and withheld the power to exercise it. While drawing attention to the number of Irishmen who had risen to high office in the Empire, he told the Commons that "the class of my fellow countrymen who clamour for the right of self government fail utterly to show the possession of these qualities which would ensure its proper use . . ."(5) If Ireland separated from England, the Irish would, like the Kilkenny cats, fight among themselves till nothing was left but their tails.

It was a speech showing how little he understood of the convictions of a majority of his countrymen. His opponents called his ideas "politically immoral," and accused him of subscribing to the view "that they should take who have the power and they should keep who they can."(6)

In between debates Arthur pestered successive governments on a range of issues from dredging of Dunmore
harbour to the burning in effigy of Judge Keogh by the
Kerry militia and the death of Richard Dickinson of the
4th Dragoon Guards who, after helping to fight a fire in
Carlow, was plied with so much whiskey by a grateful
people, that he died of "an overdose of alcohol."

He harassed the First Lord of the Admiralty unceasingly
on the Maegara affair. HMS Maegara, a transport ship,
overloaded and badly holed, had been obliged to land its
crew on a deserted island to await rescue by a Dutch
ship. Arthur had questioned its sea worthiness before it
set out on its voyage to Sidney and received dismissive
replies. He elicited facts about the sea worthiness of
other naval vessels, asked questions on the loss of church
records, on the extension of educational facilities to
girls; and on the future of the Earl of Grannard as
Lord Lieutenant in Leitrim, after he had displeased him
by chairing the tenants rights meeting at which Father
Doyle had spoken. Turning his attention to railways, he
advocated amalgamation to improve efficiency, since
there was, he complained, a director for every two
miles of track in Ireland.

Arthur firmly resisted any move towards democracy,
whether nationally or locally. He opposed the Ballot
Act which gave electors the right to a secret vote,
and dismissed moves to abolish the Grand Jury, which
was made up of local gentlemen, and replace it by
elected members. Dublin's problems of increasing debt,
and streets like ploughed fields according to season, he
attributed to the ineptitude of the "lower classes" who
ran the city's affairs to the exclusion of the gentry.(7)

In debates on religious matters he kept his own counsel.
He was "pious," but not in a denominational sense.
He voted at the outset of his parliamentary career to
preserve the established status of the Church of Ireland,
and worked hard to give a sound financial basis to the
disendowed church. He advised on the new Prayer Book
but never spoke in Parliament in defence of the Church

of Ireland. In 1879 a firmly Protestant Arthur was to be found in the unlikely company of the O'Connor Don, Parnell the Home Ruler, Mr Shaw and the wild Lord Beresford, in proposing a University Education (Ireland) Bill. He was concerned that his "Roman Catholic fellow countrymen" were denied access to university education. He told the House that to attempt to teach in a totally objective manner was impossible. It was impossible to teach the history of a nation without reference to its religion. If students could not come together in one educational establishment because of the attitudes of the religious authorities, they should be educated in a place of their choice, but come together in a common centre to sit a common examination. It was a simple remedy but one which did not commend itself to "bigots," to the Scottish members, or to the anonymous writers who accused the Bill's sponsors of disseminating error. "Who amongst us is qualified," he asked, "to pronounce his brother in error?" But despite pleas for justice and fair play, the Bill was lost.(8)

Towards the end of the 1870's the corn growing areas of the Western States of America flooded European markets with their produce, aided by improved rail and shipping connexions. Farm prices fell and the small Irish farmer was once more too poor to pay his rent. The potato crop failed, poverty ensued and evictions increased from 463 families in 1877 to 2,110 in 1880, each representing a well of misery. The Irish Relief Bill granted a million in loans to be distributed by the landlords, many of them absentees, to the poor they had evicted. At the beginning of 1880 the Duchess of Marlborough, wife of the Lord Lieutenant of Ireland, was "compelled to start Relief Funds to avert a dreadful calamity."

On the 24th March 1880 Parliament was dissolved. Disraeli, now Lord Beaconsfield, issued his election manifesto in the form of a letter to the Duke of Marlborough, calling for support to give England an ascendancy in the Councils of Europe and check the Home Rule Movement in Ireland, which he considered "scarcely less disastrous than pestilence or famine."(9)

Just as Borris had once irked Arthur, London now did. He had sat in Parliament under the third Derby-Disraeli Ministry, under the reforming first Ministry of Gladstone, which left ministers like a range of "extinct volcanoes;" and under the last Ministry of Beaconsfield which, being absorbed in foreign affairs, had failed to manage the disorderly House of Commons obstructed in its business by Parnell. Disillusioned and frustrated by the government's failure to deal with the Irish problems, Borris and RYS Eva became his havens. The "Fashionable Intelligence" column of the Carlow Sentinel noted his comings and goings. On the Eva he was free of contention, polemic, of the land questions and religion. Sailing in the Caledonian Canal, as though a thousand miles away, he noted a strange grey patch with heaving coils of a black substance and a water spout which his cousin Sarah Steel interpreted as the Loch Ness Monster. He still retained, at home, his sense of fun on the Victorian model. He organised charades and performances of scenes from Scott's novels and from Shakespeare with the Marquis of Ormonde, his cousin and Grace Osborne, Duchess of Saint Albans, a kinswoman of his mother, taking leading roles.

He remained seemingly oblivious of his handicaps. When visiting Lady de Vesci he was pleased to note after a long absence that the local station master remembered him. Only rarely did his anger betray itself. When his body servant stumbled while carrying him at Bagnelstown station, they both fell onto the track in front of the stationary engine. Never, said a passer-by, had she witnessed such a look of hatred as she then saw in Arthur Kavanagh's eyes.

On the 14th of January 1877, Walter Kavanagh came of age. The celebrations were deferred until October so that his father could be present. The Courtyard of Borris House was roofed over, and "richly decorated" and "brilliantly illuminate" with gas chandeliers.(10)

The Conservative press indulged in its customary adulation of the Kavanaghs as the son of the "popular

and esteemed Lord of the soil" reached his majority.(11)
They traced his descent once again from Milesius to the
elected kings of Leinster and the chieftains recognized
by Henry VIII, and gave him a Plantagenet ancestry
through the marriage of Cahir McArt to Elizabeth
Fitzgerald, granddaughter of the Marquis of Dorset.
They did not mention his common ancestry with the
Queen; both descended from Dermot MacMurrough;
Queen Victoria from Dermot's daughter Eva Countess
of Pembroke, the Mortimers and Edward IV; and Walter
from Dermot's son Donnel who adopted the name of
Kavanagh from the place of his fosterage Kilcavan.

At the Ball at Borris on the 9th of October family and
friends gathered. The Ormondes, were there with the
Bruens, the Alexanders, the Beresfords and the Bookeys.
The 18th Regiment from Kilkenny Barracks provided
the music and there was a novelty in the form of a
"singing quadrille." Missing was Lady Harriet, ailing
at Ballyragget, "dear Hoddy" who had died the previous
year, and the beloved Boxwell.

Arthur called on "the boys" to drink the Queen's health
and enthused over the coming of age of his heir, which
was of such importance to him and to them. Clanship
bound them together; his success was their success, his
adversity theirs. The mountains beyond, if they could
speak, would testify of the gatherings between all their
ancestors in war, victory and peace and there was no
greater jewel in a monarch's crown than his people's
love. It was again the stuff on which he had been
reared and fed as an adolescent when, in his families
absence, he had laid the foundations of his relationship
with his tenants and labourers.

It was twenty two years since he had presented Frances
to them and told them they would come to know her and
love her and value her for herself. They had welcomed
her for his sake; now she had earned her own place in
their hearts.

No one, he told them, was better placed to wish a son

every blessing, temporal and eternal, than his father. And whatever temptations the world might hold, the blood that ran in his sons veins would ensure that he did his duty and passed on to his descendants, and theirs, in unbroken love and unimpaired integrity, the trust and confidence of a happy prosperous and loving people.

Walter's reply was short and colourless. He thanked the tenants for their good wishes; some of them he knew through shooting on their lands and others he hoped to get to know. With such a father to guide and direct him and with the example of what he had done and continued to do, it would be hard to go far wrong and he pledged to follow his father's example.

Sweetman, who had attacked the Kavanaghs for their mistreatment of their tenants during Tom's minority and Robert Doynes administration, rose to challenge any of his hearers to show a single harsh act towards a tenant on the Kavanagh estates. When tenants were in difficulty, he said, Arthur "nursed" them out of it; when disease ravaged their herds he replaced them.(12)

A more reliable witness than Sweetman was Father Carey, Parish Priest of Borris. He introduced a note of realism. He spoke, he said, excluding politics, polemic and adulation, but truthfully and independently. Firstly he drew attention to Frances and her attractiveness, though it was not appropriate for a man of his calling to dwell on that. She was courageous and persevering in face of many obstacles. Like the woman in Solomon she was a good wife and her husband praised her; she was charitable in word and work and "stretched out her hand to the poor"; she had introduced lace making and encouraged temperance and helped the poor to clothe themselves through her Borris club. Arthur, said Father Carey, built houses for the poor, propped up "tottering tenants" and all that he did was free from the "stain of bigotry." If there had been bigotry Father Carey would not have been with them today. He thanked Arthur and Frances, for the way in which they treated their tenants, and he assured them that Catholics did not want ascendancy but equality. They had received "fair play" in that direction from Mr and Mrs Kavanagh, and they reigned as "uncrowned and sceptreless monarchs" in the hearts and affections of their people.(13)

17. REJECTION

The election campaign of 1880 was turbulent: land and Home Rule were the major issues; the secret ballot the most important weapon for change. There was great tenant interest in the downfall of the landlords. Many of the former were, as Arthur had pointed out in a letter to the parish priest of Borris, "heavily in debt,"(1) and a redistribution of land would solve their problems. The Land League was putting pressure on tenants not to pay rent and terrorising many who did. The downfall of the landlords would bring them relief from the dual pressure of League and Landlord.

Active in County Carlow and elsewhere for a year before the election was called was Father Ryan, curate of St Mullins. He was a Land League man and a Home Ruler. He had canvassed forcefully to convince people that with the secret ballot the landlord would have no knowledge of how they voted and consequently could not punish them for voting against him with eviction. He produced a bound booklet "The Political Services of Kavanagh and Bruen and what they have done for Carlow," and delivered it to every voter in the area who, when they opened it, found only blank pages. It was an election ploy, not strictly accurate, and designed to make Arthur and Bruen a "laughing stock."(2)

The anti-landlord, Home Rule candidates were a wealthy Scottish Liberal, Donald McFarlane and E. Dwyer Gray, Lord Mayor of Dublin. Father Ryan urged the voters to "put the sign of the cross after the names of Gray and McFarlane and leave the rest to God."(3)

Arthur and Bruen were considered to be two of the most influential Irish members of Parliament by the Conservative press, while their opponents were dismissed as a "host of carpet baggers." Gray, it was said, had never set foot in Arthur Kavanagh's "model town," while Kavanagh and Bruen were "cordially received everywhere they went and were confident of a narrow majority based on the promises of their tenants.(4)

An anti-landlord meeting was held in front of the Parish priest's house in Borris, and both McFarlane and Gray addressed it. Neither attacked Arthur, but complimented him as a landlord while falsely accusing him of voting for the Inspection of Convents Bill, designed to open up convents to the scrutiny of independent assessors. It was a measure zealously pursued by anti-Catholic groups and equally zealously deplored by Catholics. The Lady Mayoress of Dublin, spoke to the voters from a window of the priest's house; the same priest who had lavished praise on Arthur at his son's coming of age a little over two years earlier. Gray and McFarlane claimed, with some justification, to be men of issues rather than personalities. Their opponents regarded them as men hiding behind "petticoats and priests" to address a "motley collection" of non-voters."(5)

Arthur arrived at Borris station at 4.45 the same after-noon and was met by a "large and enthusiastic crowd." He spoke to the voters from his horse in the gateway of the Lodge, basing his appeal on his past record and past criteria. He had not changed his principles; he had denounced capricious evictions, allowed compensation for improvements before legislation required it and had encouraged education and supported the amendment, though not the abolition of the undemocratic Grand Jury System. Arthur told the voters he saw no cause for them to think their confidence in him had been misplaced. He nailed the lie about voting for the Convents Inspection Bill, and told them he had earlier that day met the Catholic Bishop Walshe and gained the impression the bishop did not support the Home Rulers. At this point the Catholic curates began a counter demonstration a hundred yards away, trying to drown Arthur's voice.

On the day of the election he rode to Kilkenny to cast his vote for Lord Arthur Butler; on his way home, as he dipped and rose on the undulating road, he saw that "The mountains and hilltops of Kilkenny and Carlow were

ablaze."(6)   So often this had been a sign of victory
and celebration for the Kavanagh's over the centuries.
From the top of the hill as he entered Borris, he could
see the fires more clearly; but as he rode along the
demesne wall past his model cottages with Frances' rose
bushes at the door, he was met not by cheers but by
jeers and catcalls.   The crowds were hostile.   The fires
were celebrating not his victory but his defeat, and "the
Cripple Kavanagh"(7) as they called him, was burning in
a monstrous effigy. He couldn't believe what he saw
and then turned his back on them and rode into the
safety of the demesne.

" . . . these were the men whom he had loaded with
benefit, on whose families he had spent thousands of
pounds without asking or expecting interest, to whose
families in sickness or health, in prosperity or adversity,
he had shown the most unwearied kindness; with whom
he had lived and worked for a quarter of a century on
terms of the greatest confidence and cordiality."(8)

Frances acknowledged, despite her reservations in 1862,
that Arthur's years in Parliament had been his happiest.
She was away from Borris when news of his defeat came
and she wrote him a consoling letter. His reply survives:

11th April 1880

"Many thanks for your dear letter.

"It would be folly to deny that the blow is a sharp
one, but to me it was not unexpected, for I always
felt how hollow was the ground we stood upon.

"The sharpest part of it is the belief that is forced
upon me that the majority of my own men broke
their promises to me.   My confidence in them is
gone, and a great interest and pleasure in home-life
gone with it.

"That is the poisoned stab. If I could have believed
them true, the actual defeat would be easy to bear,
because I have nothing that I can see to be ashamed
of in it.   But to have to look forward to passing the

rest of my life among them is almost more than I can do.

"I do not think more than forty of my fellows gave me a vote. But there is no good in brooding over it, and I must guard against the natural impulse to resent it, which God alone can help one to do.

"Do not, my darling, fret yourself for me. I look upon defeat as God's will, and try to take it as such. That makes it lighter than I could have believed.

"The sting that rankles is the treachery and deceit of my own men - 'my own familiar friends in whom I trusted' - but that feeling must be choked. I wish I could say or do something to cheer your own dear self. Believe what is the real truth: that is all for the best. It must be, as it was ordered so."(9)

Arthur's trust in "his" people, perhaps even in people in general was damaged. Since the annual celebrations at Borris House when he was a youth, they had protested their loyalty to the Kavanaghs, and he in particular had been conscious of historic bonds between them. One great bond had been broken when his father conformed to the Established Church, a second when the "unhappy connexion" with the alien Protestant Ascendancy had been forged by his parents' marriage and his mother's arrival as mistress of Borris. All these years they had, he thought, been insincere, bearing a grudge, taking all they could get; and when the secret ballot broke the landlord's hold, they turned him out.

He had failed to understand his people's desire to be Irish, in Ireland, and failed to understand that for them Ireland was not a fragment of England. He had failed to understand that they did not want good landlords but no landlords at all, particularly those associated with a "foreign power." He had grasped that the growth of democracy meant the end of the Ascendancy and had resisted it.

In his early years at Celbridge and at Borris, what he felt as rejection by his ever absent mother, had left him desolate, and he had forged bonds with the tenants who felt equally deserted when the "big house" was empty. When she sent him out to roam around the world he had turned it to his advantage and became the admiration of his peers. Years of appreciation of his courage and determination had followed from all quarters, but when his people turned him out it was unexpected and he was desolate, bitter and angry. He felt physically ill when he met his tenants and the local villagers. He was coldly courteous and contemptuous of what he considered to be their deceit. He couldn't bear the thought of living the rest of his life among them.

After Eton and Christchurch, and now a Captain in the Royal Irish Rifles, Walter came home to learn about Estate Management. Charles had left Harrow and was at Sandhurst, and young Arthur, his father's favourite, was soon to leave Dartmouth and take up a Commission in the Royal Navy. It was the names of the boys and their sisters which now figured in the guest lists at County Balls and functions at the Carlow Club House. Arthur and Frances contented themselves with occasional week-ends with their Butler relatives at Kilkenny Castle, from which they could ride in the Parkland, dally in the Long Gallery or look out over the medieval jewel of a city.

Soon after his electoral defeat he was appointed as the Queen's Lieutenenat in Carlow, raising him, for some, to the most important rank in the County; for others, identifying him still further with the English Crown.

In the new Parliament, Gladstone was aware that there would be no peace in Ireland until the land question was settled, and introduced a new Land Bill amending the Act of 1870 in the tenants favour. The Lords rejected it and the Government acquiesced promising a new bill in the following year. The gap was filled by the appointment of a Commission to investigate the working of recent Land Legislation in Ireland.

On July 29th 1880 the "Trusty and Well Beloved Arthur MacMurrough Kavanagh Esq"(10) was appointed by the Queen, along with Baron Dowse, Charles Owen O'Connor and Mr Shaw, to be a member of the Commission, headed by Lord Bessborough.

As a member of the Commission Arthur began to travel throughout Ireland, hearing evidence of the plight of tenants and landlords and the activities of the Land League. Founded in 1879 the League, headed by Parnell the Protestant landlord from Wicklow, urged tenants to pay a fair rent, which was one a tenant could afford according to the times, and to "hold firm to their home-steads."(11) The League used violence against landlords, their agents and anyone who rented land from which others had been evicted. Parnell disliked violence and advocated other methods, urging the populace to shun those who opposed the League's activities, in the streets, at the shop counter, even in the church, where they were to treat them as lepers.

The Bessborough Commission sat in the Railway Hotel in Galway in mid-October 1880. Arthur questioned Mr Charles Cunningham-Boycott, who told him that a mob had come to his house on the shores of Loch Mask, which he rented from Lord Erne, and ordered off every-one in his employment. No one would work for him. "I cannot get my potatoes dug or my hay saved." he said, "I cannot get my corn threshed nor my mangolds cut, and after this frost my mangolds will be worthless."(12) Boycott and Lord Erne were not the worst of landlords. They had in the previous year reduced rents, but would not bow to further pressure from the Land League, and Boycott was driven out of Mayo, while his name became a household word. Arthur was a patient listener to the witnesses. He pressed a Mr Blake on what, in his opinion, was the smallest holding a man without any other means of support could decently exist upon. He prodded William Halliday of Bushy Park on the injustice of evicting in the Famine years. He listened in silence to Patrick Noon's account of how eighteen tenants lived on forty acres with dependants totalling nearly two hundred.(13)

On December the 2nd, while staying at Bushy Park as a guest of Halliday, Arthur wrote to E W Forster, the Chief Secretary for Ireland, expressing the view that "the people of Ireland should be made to obey the law, "before any conciliatory land legislation was introduced." (14) As a descendant of Huguenot emigres he was haunted by fears of another massacre of St Bartholomew, advising the Chief Secretary that the condition of the country was worse than at any time since the rebellion of 1798. He did not anticipate a general uprising, but was certain that some parts of the country were prepared for it. He believed a settlement of the land issue was essential for peace, but concessions only led to demands for more. He recommended that when Parliament met in the new year the Queen's Speech should contain a warning that the Government would not consider the Land Question until order was restored. He believed that the suspension of Habeus Corpus, though regrettable, would have a magical effect.

On the 24th of January 1881, the first day of the new session of Parliament, Forster introduced the Protection of Persons (Ireland) Bill, enabling the Lord Lieutenant to arrest by warrant any persons suspected of treasonable intentions, intimidation and incitement to violate the law.

When the Bessborough Report was published, Arthur could not accept it in its entirety and submitted his own independent report. From the evidence he had heard, he believed that the majority of the properties of the larger landlords were "properly and humanely" managed; rents were low and rarely raised, and evictions, except for non payment of rent, were few. He believed that rent was at the root of most grievances; that the Land Act of 1870 did not give sufficient protection against unjust raising of rents, and he approved of arbitration where landlord and tenant could not agree. He was firmly against further extension of the right of tenants to sell their holdings, and this last issue was the major difference between himself and other members of the Commission.

SACKVILLE STREET CLUB.

DUBLIN.

10-1-89

My dear Ashbourne

I recd a note from
Mr Balfour last night in:
forming me that His Excellency
had been kind enough to
appoint young Bowen to the
vacant office of Resident
Magistrate I have of course
written to His Ex to thank
him but I know that my
chief thanks are due to you.
for without your most
kind interest I do not

Facsimile of letter from Arthur Kavanagh to Lord Ashbourne

believe he same wd have
got so you must allow
me to write a line to thank
you most sincerely for
yr kindness
I thought I shd have seen
you at Privy Council
today or I wd have
written sooner
Believe me with many thanks
Yrs sincerely
Arthur Kavanagh

Gladstone introduced his second Land Bill on the 7th April and in his speech paid tribute to "Mr Kavanagh." "I will not mention his name," Gladstone told the House, "without saying that he is one of the ablest, if not the ablest gentleman coming from Ireland, I have ever known among the party opposite. Besides his ability, he is a man of independent mind and I do not scruple to call him - making allowances for his starting point - a man of liberal and enlightened feelings."(15)

On April 14th Arthur wrote thanking Gladstone for "your very kind mention of me in your speech introducing the Land Bill. It is a compliment which I never expected and it is on that account more valued." Gladstone's instruction for a reply are written on the back "received with much gratification and that opinion recently expressed is not of recent formation."(16)

The new Land Act allowed tenants to sell their interests to the highest bidder and set up land Courts to fix the rents by judicial process, recognizing dual ownership between landlord and tenant. For Arthur it was too radical, allowing tenants to manipulate the highest price and giving the landlord too little control over incoming tenants, while striking at the root of the landlords' case by confirming dual ownership. The Land League also disapproved of it because they did not want improved tenants' rights, but the abolition of landlords. The Act did not bring peace to Ireland. The Land League, which renewed its agitation for the withholding of rents, was dissolved by the Government and its leaders imprisoned. Their subsequent release led to the Chief Secretary's resignation and the appointment of Lord Frederick Cavendish as Chief Secretary in Ireland. When Lord Frederick was murdered in Pheonix Park by a group of conspirators, further coercion followed.

More and more Arthur came to believe that a peasant proprietorship, giving the people a stake in the land, was the only solution.

The year 1882 was dominated by domestic as well

as political matters. In July Eva Frances, Arthur's
elder daughter, married Cecil Alexander, son of the
Archbishop of Armagh and Mrs Alexander author of
the book of "Hymns for Little Children" which included
"Once in Royal David's City", "There is a green hill
far away" and "All things bright and beautiful." Arthur
approved of the philosophy expressed in the latter:

> "The rich man in his castle
> The poor man at his gate
> God made them high and lowly
> And ordered their estate."

Less happy was news of young Arthur, now a Lieutenant
in the Royal Navy. Dartmouth, he had told his grandmother in a letter thanking her for the gift of a pocket
book, was "an awful place." Nothing ever went on and he
couldn't wait to get back to Borris where he and Walter
would be in their "glory," and while the family were away
for Easter they would of course go over to Ballyragget
to see her.(17)

Young Arthur's antipathy to Dartmouth may have been
a young man's dissatisfaction with a place where nothing
ever happened, rather than with his chosen career; for
even after two bouts of bronchitis had convinced him
that naval doctors were "idiots," he wrote to his father
expressing disappointment at missing his ship as a result.
Letters from the South Atlantic brought to Borris details
of the partridge shooting around Montevideo and, like
his grandmother on her Middle Eastern tours, he noted
the price of beef and mutton. Everything except meat
was "fearfully expensive."(18)

By June 1881 he was making it clear to his mother that
he wanted to leave the Navy and to go into commerce.
When his father learned of this he wrote a letter which
was a mixture of anger, sorrow, blackmail and encouragement. He warned his son of the difficulties of going into
"trade". "I must say, from what I know of you, you like
association with gentlemen of your own class, and you
have that in the navy more than any other profession."(19)

Trade, he warned, was precarious and remuneration poor. With his talent young Arthur would reach, in the navy, a status trade could never give. He was sorry and grieved by the thought of his son leaving the service which would "quench" the great hope "which he had in him."

In the course of the letter, Arthur's plan for his son unfolded. The ambition which he had "indulged" and "in a foolishly strong way," was "to pull the family out of the sort of oblivion and obscurity into which, certainly since my father's death, it has lapsed. With that object I have worked constantly against no small difficulties both pecuniary and others." He made clear that his future hopes for the family lay not with his heir but with his second son, and he told him "When you made your start and gained your triumph I thought, well thank God I have got one to make and perhaps leave a name and now all I ask you, and I will say no more, is to stick to your profession and to do your best." Young Arthur could not resist the pressure and the plea of his "affectionate father" who pinned such hopes on him. (20)

Lieutenant Arthur Kavanagh was a popular crew member. "Charley Beresford," now Admiral Lord Charles, recorded how during one of his bouts of bronchitis, he refused to go sick before completing the discharge of torpedoes from HMS Vernon. The chest problems, however, grew worse and by Autumn 1882 he was too ill to continue in the navy and was brought back to England, believing that all he needed to restore his health, was a trip to Madeira. In November when he arrived at his parents' house at 62 Cadogan Place in London, he was able to propel himself in his wheel chair; three weeks later he could not move without help. Arthur and Frances accepted that their son was dying but decided, on the advice of their doctor, to humour him. If he thought a trip to Madeira would help, they would go along with it. On November 20th Frances, Walter and young Arthur boarded the Drummond Castle at Blackwall. Arthur watched them go and then returned to Cadogan Place to write to his "dearest mother."

"So he is gone," he told her and, "of course I shall never see him again. Poor Fan and Walter are with him and a sad task they have for it can only be to see him die." His sufferings were "immense" and he confided in his mother that he wished God would take his son, for he couldn't bear the thought of him sitting up in a close cabin unable to lie down.(21) Two days later Arthur telegraphed the news of his son's death to Lady Harriet. The boy had liked his cabin and had slept better. He had awakened at 4 am on Tuesday in no pain, but rather cold. They had put bottles to his feet to warm him and then he died.

Arthur's grief turned to an irrational anger against the people of Borris. He would not allow those in whom he had placed such trust and who, he believed, had betrayed him, to share his grief. He wrote to Lady Harriet, explaining, "I have selected a pretty spot near the little church in the Woking cemetery that I can always see as I pass up and down the line. I felt a loathing against bringing the poor fellow home (although St Mullin was a natural place to lay him) where he would be followed by a crowd of howling hypocrites, whose pretended grief would be measured by their hat bands and who would as soon have cursed him if the humour took them. How changed from the old times when one used to believe their professions."(22)

There were consoling letters of condolence from young Arthur's shipmates and tributes to his sense of duty, his splendid discipline and his amiable qualities. Charles Beresford wrote, "I had the greatest affection for him. He was one of the best officers in the navy and a real loss to the country."(23)

If Arthur felt remorse at having brought pressure on his son to remain in the navy, it was passed over in silence. He consoled himself with his son's readiness for death, while Frances busied herself planning the erection of a window to her son's memory in the family chapel.

18. THE DECLINING YEARS

Denied the platform of the Imperial Parliament,
Arthur found other channels through which he sought
to influence Irish affairs. He wrote papers and letters,
gave interviews and sat on interminable committees.

Taking his cue from Sir George Trevelyan, who had
spoken of two Irelands, that of the intelligent, well
educated, law abiding and prosperous and that of the
ignorant, disloyal and poverty stricken, Arthur wrote his
own paper. The division, as he saw it, was not between
Tory and Whig, Catholic and Protestant, landlord and
dispossessed but between loyal and disloyal. The loyal
included the "poorer grades;" small tenant farmers, shop-
keepers and tradesmen, all tired of the intimidation,
turmoil and misery brought by political agitators. The
disloyal included both educated and uneducated, believer
and atheist, cleric and layman, capitalist and communist,
all united by the common bond of hatred for the British
Crown. While Trevelyan saw the "disloyal" Ireland as the
smaller of the two groups, Arthur saw it as the larger,
"cowardly, dishonest and violent, brought up in treason
from their cradles and convinced by experience that
agitation paid." Their success, he believed, would lead
to civil war, as the North would never submit to rule
by the other Provinces.(1)

It was a prophetic paper but showed no sign of insight
into why large numbers of Irish men and women felt
as they did. It ignored seven hundred years of what
the Irish saw as "foreign domination," brought about by
Arthur's own ancestors; it ignored the displacement of
the native Irish landowners in favour of Scottish and
English settlers, the exclusion of the Catholic Irish
from the right to inherit, the right to exercise their
religion, the right to hold commissions in the Armed
Forces and the right to enter the professions.

The events of the mid 1880s alarmed the Ascendancy.

Gladstone's Reform Bill added an estimated two million voters to the electoral registers. Arthur's cousin, Sarah, forgetting their own descent from the Ballyshannon publican, railed against the granting of the vote to the "illiterate peasant class" which the priests would place at Parnell's disposal, "flooding Parliament with publicans, petty tradesmen, and adventurers."(2)

With rumours that the Viceroy Lord Spencer, who was seen to be upholding British authority in Ireland like Gordon in Kartoum, was to be removed; with signs of an alliance between Tories and Parnellites and with both Tories and Liberals seeming to pander to Irish extremists, the loyal Irish took fright.

An enraged Arthur wrote, from the Carlton Club, five pages of black angry script setting out his feelings. When Lady Rosebury, wife of the Foreign Secretary, forwarded them to Gladstone she thought it prudent to acknowledge, "I fear they (Arthur's views) are very violent." Gladstone thanked her and promised to "examine them with interest."(3)

In his paper Arthur claimed that Ireland had never been in a more unsettled state; trade, was paralysed, confidence in law and order gone, and civil contracts worthless. Ironically the descendant of he who had harassed Richard II's troops in Ireland, complained that the Queen's writ no longer ran in parts of the country.

Arthur saw the British Constitution as being as near perfect as was possible but it would not work with the Irish, who were "excitable and reared in disloyalty," particularly as politicians had failed to give any firm leadership. "Love of power and desire for place have penetrated mighty minds," he wrote. The "sacred trust" of the direction of a great nation had been used for the furtherance of personal ambition; words had been eaten, pledges broken. The Conservatives, he said, had shrunk from coercion, which the Irish would have welcomed, as a means of liberating them from terror; especially as they lacked the moral courage to resist terror themselves. The future of Ireland depended on a reinforcement of law and order and he begged that if the Union was not to be maintained, loyal citizens be informed so that they might escape with their lives.(4)

Gladstone chose to ignore this emotive assessment of the Irish situation and introduced a Home Rule Bill, which was perceived as virtual repeal of the Union. A complementary Land Bill gave tenants the option of buying out landlords through a government sponsored scheme. The measures failed and the Tories again took office.

On July 14th 1885 Lady Harriet died at Ballyragget Lodge, her home since Arthur's marriage. She was, according to her friends, "a woman of high culture and unusual artistic power" who had spent her later years "doing good to everyone who came within her refining influence." She had suffered a "calm decay."(5)

A hundred carriages followed the hearse from the beautifully proportioned eighteenth century house beside the river Nore and through the model village reconstructed in her lifetime. The local Court suspended its sitting and the curious lined the route. As her coffin paused, children were told how, as a young woman, she had erected a statue of the Blessed Virgin in the ballroom at Ballyragget, and how revellers had desecrated it by cutting off the hands; when Lady Harriet's son was born, he had neither arms nor legs. A moment or two later a carriage carrying that son passed by bearing witness, so they thought, to the truth of the tale.

As the cortege passed through Kilkenny, the Grand Jury assembled to pay their respects, while others murmured that she had been cursed by a beggar for refusing him alms. In Bagnalstown, children were told that Lady Harriet had once baked a cake in the shape of the Virgin and Child, and when serving it, had first cut the arms and legs of the infant Christ.

The body of the daughter of the Earl of Clancarty, wife

of "the last Chieftain and first heretic of his race," and mother of the "Cripple Kavanagh," lay in state in the chapel at Borris House for one day. The next morning, escorted by the mounted tenantry, the cortege left for St Mullins. Crowds packed the steep streets. "Memories of kindly words and deeds and the tears of those she had befriended in the dark hours of desolation and poverty welled up." The procession escorted Lady Harriet's body into "the old Abbey - there to rest in sure and certain hope till the morning of the resurrection."(6) "Kind Hearts", said the Carlow Sentinel, "are more than coronets and simple faith than Norman blood."(7)

Lady Harriet's death was followed by that of Boxwell and of Mary Conolly, Arthur's friend since childhood. His swearing in as a Privy Councillor was overshadowed by the diagnosis of diabetes. "No one who knew him only in later years could realise what he was before disappointment first, and failing health afterwards, robbed him of the bright spirits of early manhood."(8)

Walter married in 1887, acting as High Sheriff and Magistrate, as his father had done in earlier times. Although ailing, Arthur redoubled his efforts on behalf of the landlords and against the agitators.

In an interview with the New York World, Arthur explained how the landlords had countered the Land League's policy of pressurising tenants into refusing rent, by setting up the Land Corporation - sometimes known as Kavanagh's scheme. The League and its supporters regarded Arthur as the "brains of the Landlord's Party." (9) A first move of the Corporation was to give armed protection to the poorer landlords whose fortunes had declined since the Famine, and who were now being ruined by the refusal of tenants to pay rent. A more subtle move was to have damages for non payment of rent and malicious injury at the hands of the League's supporters, paid out of local taxes, to which tenant farmers contributed. This policy led to the undermining of tenant farmers' support for the League. Landlords were encouraged to appeal to the Courts against settlements which they considered too low, and were given financial backing by the Land Corporation to do so. When the League put pressure on local people not to take up tenancies of farms from which others had been evicted, the Derelict Land Trust was formed by the landlords to purchase, reclaim and work the land.

The Papal condemnation of the League's activities on the grounds that they prevented tenants from entering lawful contracts, and of boycotting on the grounds that it was against Christian charity, was a victory for the Landlords, while the reduction of rents by the Land Commission was a defeat.

Arthur's diary for 1889 survives. In the early months he was preoccupied by the "Ponsonby Affair." Charles Talbot Ponsonby had lost almost £25,000 in rent, owed his solicitors £5,000, and was about to sell his estates for a pittance, when a syndicate of wealthy landlords operating "Kavanagh's Scheme" bought him out for a good price, evicting non-paying tenants and making them a drain on the League's funds until it gave in. It was an example of the Land Corporation at its most effective.

Though troubled by chest pains and bad toothache Arthur spent his time "tackling" his increasing correspondence. Some days he wrote forty letters. As and when he could he relaxed with his family in London, dining with his daughter Eva and her husband, driving out with Frances and his grandson "little Cecil Alexander." Some days Frances dropped him at the Carlton Club and then went on to shop at the "Haymarket Co-op;" other days they shopped together at the "Army and Navy Co-op." On Sundays they went to the Chapel of the Royal Hospital which was around the corner from their London home, 19 Tedworth Square.

On February 24th Arthur travelled back to Ireland on the Mail train, and was glad to have a carriage to himself. Two days later when the snow lay thick across the hills, he took the early train from Borris to Carlow, had breakfast at the Club and then went on to the Courthouse for the swearing in of the Grand Jury. He remained at the Court until both the fiscal and criminal business were completed, taking the train back at 2.30 pm.

Despite a "seedy cough" and a North East wind he was off to London again on March 16th. It was a "lovely night" and he sat on deck until 4 am, arriving at Tedworth Square twelve hours later. He found it cooler than in Ireland; his "rheumatism" in the chest troubled him and after a short period of letter writing he had to "knock off." He felt at times "wretchedly hot" and "wretchedly good for nothing" and his weight was down to 7 stone 5lbs.(10) After a few days sailing in the Channel he returned to Ireland and another round of meetings.

He noted Walter and his daughter-in-law Helen's comings and goings and their late returns with some disapproval, and when his life-long acquaintance Sweetman visited him he wrote, "old humbug." In another entry he wrote, "Had a line from Charlie (his second son) in pencil written on board steamer 'The Nile' - saying goodbye!"(11)

On the eighth of June, with the Steeles and Cecil Alexander and three maids, he took a boat down river to St Mullins. They spent a day, reminiscent of many earlier happy outings, at his small cottage in the woods, broke an oar on the journey and arrived back home by 6 pm.

His frequent visits to Dublin, for the meetings of his numerous committees, continued until he left Ireland for Cowes at the end of July. He had a splendid time meeting old friends, The Duke of Westminster, Lord Dufferin, Grace Osborne, Duchess of St. Albans, the Ormondes and Lord Stafford. The Kaiser arrived at Spithead on 1st August, escorted by twelve German warships. The Naval Review took place on the 5th of August, and on board the Royal Yacht, Queen Victoria handed her grandson the commission of Admiral of the Fleet. Charlie Beresford, Admiral and protégé of the Prince of Wales and Arthur's life long friend, came

on board his yacht to see him, and he was delighted.
The Duchess of St Albans did not arrive, and he was
disappointed.

At the end of Cowes week he sailed for Holland. Most
of the time it rained but on the 31st August, "the sun
came out and grilled us."(12)   Arthur's writing was
deteriorating. By the end of October his printing was
that of a child. He repeated himself, crossed out and
began again and spilled ink on the pages. On the 9th
October the Carlow Sentinel told readers that Arthur
had "passed a very restless night." On the 11th he
"had a good night not withstanding the liquorice powder"
and on the 12th his doctor reassured him that his chest
pains were indigestion; he went down to dinner and
"felt much better." On 17th October, "I thought I had
a fair night but was told I had a very bad one . . . felt
very drowsy." On 12th November he went for a drive
after lunch, calling at his club where he was weighed -
just six stone eleven and a half ounces. From this point
a firmer hand took over until entries in the diary ceased
on the 4th of December with "Lord de Vesci called."

Arthur died at 4 am on Christmas morning at Tedworth
Square. His daughter Eva was at his bedside. The cause
of death was given as "diabetes of unknown duration"
and "phithisis pulmonalis, left lung, duration unknown."
(13) The "rheumatism" in the chest turned out to be
tuberculosis.

The news of his death was announced in the Carlow
Sentinel and Kilkenny Moderator on pages edged with
black, and on the following Sunday the congregation in
St Canice's Cathedral at Kilkenny, with the strains of
the Dead March echoing in their ears, heard the Bishop
of Ossory sketch his life; a great and good man, and
a tower of strength whose unique position by ancestry
and birth linked him to the history of Ireland; "he held
rank besides which most patents of nobility seemed to
be things of yesterday." His voice, said the bishop, had
been listened to with respect in the Imperial Councils;
he was a formidable but fair opponent, a loving husband

and tender father, "kindliness and consideration were as natural to him as the sunshine."(14) A more valuable testimony came from his enemies. "He was born without arms or legs - merely stumps - and apart from politics, his life was a noble example of indeterminable courage and triumph over physical disability that would daunt a weaker man."(15)

Denied his wish of dying among "his people," his body was brought back to the chapel at Borris House now hung with black, and his friends filed passed his oak coffin covered by a purple velvet pall. The fourth of January was a warm day. The shops in the village of Borris were closed, the streets empty and the populace deprived of the spectacle of a funeral cortege on its way to the burial ground of the kings at St Mullins. The coffin was carried down the steps of the chapel and placed in a hearse waiting in front of the House. Frances and her daughters entered the solitary carriage; Walter, Osborne, Henry Bruen, Cecil Alexander, Lord Ormonde, Pack-Beresford and the Pakenhams walked behind. The short procession turned its back on the village, taking a path through the demesne under "a glorious sun beguiling the birds into believing it was not winter."(16) Gradually the fields and terraces turned black with onlookers standing in silence.

Against the backdrop of Mount Leinster, with its "nebulous crown" unchanged through the centuries of Kavanagh rule, the procession reached the brook where Arthur had so often fished. "Loyal tenants" lifted the coffin from the hearse and carried it into the fields; and beside the ruined chapel of Ballycopigan, where he had so often "axed," laid it in a grave lined with moss.

BIBLIOGRAPHY

Bence-Jones, Mark: Twilight of the Ascendancy,
    Constable, 1987

Beresford, Lord Charles: Memoirs,
    Methuen & Co. Ltd, 1914

Burke: Irish Family Records

Complete Peerage: London, 1936

Creevy Papers: ed. John Gore, Batsford, 1963

Granville, Harriet Countess of: Letters,
    ed. The Hon F Leveson-Gower, Longmans Green & Co, 1894

History and Antiquities of the Diocese of Ossory

Keller, Werner: The Bible as History,
    Hodder & Stoughton, 1980

Kee, Robert: Ireland, a History,
    Book Club Associates, 1980

Longford, Elizabeth: Victoria RI,
    Wiedenfeld & Nicholson, 1964

Longford, Elizabeth: Wellington, Years of The Sword,
    Weidenfeld & Nicholson, 1969

Longford, Elizabeth: Wellington, Pillar of State,
    Weidenfeld & Nicholson, 1972

MacCarthy, M J: Handicaps; Six Studies,
    Longmans Green & Co, 1936

McCormick, D: The Incredible Mr Kavanagh,
    Putnam & Co. 1960

Medical Directory of Ireland 1843

Simmington: Transplantation to Connacht 1654-8,
    Irish University Press

Simms, J.G: The Williamite Confiscations

Steele, Sarah L: The Rt Hon Arthur MacMurrough Kavanagh,
    MacMillan, 1891

Woodham Smith, Cecil: The Great Hunger,
    Hamish Hamilton, 1962

Wilson, Robert: Life & Times of Queen Victoria,
    Cassel & Co Ltd, 1891

PUBLISHED PAPERS

Irish Family Treasures,   Eason & Son Ltd, Dublin 1985

St Mullins, St Michael's Tombstone Inscriptions,
    St Mullins Muintir Na Tire

The Kavanagh Kings, W V Hadden. CCCL

Thomas Kavanagh MP and his Political Contemporaries,
    P J Kavanagh. CCCL

Three Monasteries, E T Brophy. CCCL

The Parish of Ballinasloe, Rev P Egan. GCL(B)

Ballinasloe, T Maclochlain. GCL(B)

Castletown, Co Kildare, Craig, Glin & Cornforth. IGS,
    reprinted from Country Life, March-April 1969

The Fall of the Clan Kavanagh, Rev J Hughes. NLI

Blackwood's Edinburgh Magazine, 1891

The Lancet, 1891

Composition of The Galway Gentry, Patrick Melvin,
    Irish Genealogist. IGRS 1986

The Kavanagh's 1400-1700, Nichols,
    Irish Genealogist. IGRS 1977

MANUSCRIPTS

Pedigree of the ancient illustrious noble and princely
    House of Kavanagh, Burke 1817, Borris House, County Carlow

The Kavanagh Papers, Borris House, County Carlow

The Kavanagh Papers, National Library of Ireland

Letters of Lady Louisa Conolly,
    in the care of Mrs Lena Boylan, Celbridge

O'Leary Manuscript, The Political Services of Bruen & Kavanagh
    and what they have done for Carlow, CCL

The Gladstone Papers, British Library

REFERENCES

The following abbreviations are used:

BL	British Libray
CCCL	Carloviana, Carlow County Libray
CCL	Carlow County Library
GCL(B)	Galway County Library, (Ballinasloe)
GRO	General Register Office, London, WC2
IGRS	Irish Geneological Research Society
IGS	The Irish Georgian Society, (Castledown)
KP	Kavanagh Papers, (National Library of Ireland)
NLI	National Library of Ireland
NGI	National Gallery of Ireland

CHAPTER 1

1   The Lancet, 14th March 1891.

2   Thomas Kavanagh and his Political Contemporaries, P J Kavanagh. CCCL.

3   The Kavanagh Kings, W.V. Hadden. CCCL.

4   The Irish Genealogist, IRGS. 1977 p445.

5   History and Antiquities of The Diocese of Ossory. CCL.

6   The Parish of Ballinasloe, P Egan p179. GCL(B).

7   Memoir of the Le Poer Trench Family, Hodges Foster & Co, Dublin, 1874.

8   The Parish of Ballinasloe, P Egan p133. GCL(B).

9   The Creevy Papers, ed. John Gore, Batsford 1963.

10 Lady Louisa Conolly to her sister, 9th September 1771. IGS.

11 Richard Earl of Cancarty, The Complete Peerage.

12 Wellington to Lord Clancarty, 6th June 1822. Wellington Pillar of State, Elizabeth Longford.

13 Harriet Countess Granville to Lady Morpeth, 1st March 1824.

14 Dutton's Statistical Survey of County Galway, 1824 p331.

15 The Parish of Ballinasloe, P Egan. GCL(B).

16 Harriet Countess Granville to Lady Morpeth, 1st March 1824.

17 Lady Louisa Conolly, 28th November 1771. IGS.

CHAPTER 2

1 Francis Boxwell to Sir Philip Crampton, McCormick p12.

2 Mrs Andrew MacMurrough Kavanagh to the author, Borris, 1986.

3 The Lancet, 14th March 1891.

4 Kathleen O'Shea to the author, Drumgriffin, 1986.

5 MacCarthy p63.

6 Francis Boxwell to Sir Philip Crampton, McCormick p20.

7 Steele p8.

8 Francis Boxwell to Lady Harriet, KP 6316 P7157.

9 The Kavanagh Kings, H.V. Haddon. CCCL.

10 Mary Dundan O'Leary to Rev Sean O'Leary,
letter to the author, 25th April 1986.

11 Lady Louisa Le Poer Trench, McCormick p32.

12 MacCarthy p64.

13 Francis Boxwell to Lady Harriet Kavanagh,
McCormick p32-3.

14 Lady Harriet Kavanagh, McCormick p38.

15 John O'Leary Manuscript, The Political Services
of Bruen and Kavanagh and what they have done
for Carlow, 24th November 1941. CCL.

16 Thomas Kavanagh MP 1767-1837 and his Political
Contemporaries. CCCL.

17 Carlow Sentinel, 7th January 1837.

18 ibid.

CHAPTER 3

1 Lord Clancarty to Charles Doyne, 17th March 1837.
KP 6316 P7157

2 Lord Clancarty to Charles Doyne, 19th April 1837.

3 ibid.

4 Lord Clancarty to Charles Doyne, 25th March 1837.
ibid.

5 Lord Clancarty to Charles Doyne, 19th April 1837.
ibid.

6 Arthur Kavanagh to Lady Harriet Kavanagh,
Miscellaneous childhood letters, Borris House.

7 Castletown, County Kildare, M Craig and the
Knight of Glin. IGS 1969.

8   Lady Louisa Conolly, letters 9th September and 28th September 1771. IGS.

9   Steele p8.

10 ibid p11.

11 Arthur Kavanagh, Miscellaneous childhood letters, Borris House.

12 Carlow Sentinel, 13th November 1841.

13 Thomas Kavanagh 1676-1837, P J Kavanagh.

CHAPTER 4

1   McCormick p53.

2   Arthur Kavanagh to Lady Harriet Kavanagh, Miscellaneous childhood letters, Borris House.

3   ibid.

4   Carlow Sentinel 1st June 1844.

5   Master A. Kavanagh and Miss Harriet Kavanagh to Lady Harriet Kavanagh, Miscellaneous childhood letters, Borris House.

6   Carlow Sentinel, 16th November 1844.

7   ibid. 8th February 1845.

8   ibid.

9   ibid. 26th July 1845.

10 Lord Charles Beresford Memoirs, chapter XV.

11 Carlow Sentinel, 1st November 1845.

12 ibid.

13 MacCormick, p49.

14 Lady de Vesci to Mary MacCarthy, MacCarthy p69.

CHAPTER 5

1   McCormick p59.

2   MacCarthy pp 72-73.

3   Lady Harriet Kavanagh, Journal of a Tour in the Middle East, 3rd. October 1846. KP N6315 P7156.

4   ibid. November 1846.

5   McCormick p60.

6   ibid. p61.

7   Woodham Smith p183.

8   Exodus Ch 15, v 27.

9   ibid. Ch 16, v 13-15.

10   Keller p 131.

11   McCormick p64.

12   Arthur Kavanagh to Charles Kavanagh, 27th May 1847.
     KP N6315 P7156.

13   ibid.

14   McCormick p68.

15   Arthur Kavanagh, 26th May 1847.   KP N6315 P7156.

16   Arthur Kavanagh, McCormick   p62.

17   Arthur Kavanagh to Charles Kavanagh, 26 May 1847. KP.

18   Lady Harriet Kavanagh to Lady Louisa le Poer Trench,
     McCormick p67.

19   Lady Harriet Kavanagh to Lady Louisa undated.
     KP N6315 P7156.

20   Arthur Kavanagh to Rev Ralph Morton,
     30th October 1947. KP ibid.

21   Lady Harriet Kavanagh to Lord and Lady Clancarty,
     28th December 1847. KP ibid.

22   ibid.

23   Lady Harriet Kavanagh to Lady Louisa,
     11th December 1847. KP ibid.

24   Lady Harriet Kavanagh to Lord Clancarty,
     28th December 1847. KP ibid.

25   McCormick p63.

26   Lady Harriet Kavanagh, 6th January 1848.
     KP N6315 P7156.

27   Rev Ralph Morton, 10th April 1848. KP ibid.

28   Carlow Sentinel, 20th April 1849.

29   ibid. 6th May 1849.

30   ibid. 27th May 1849.

31   ibid.

CHAPTER 6

1   Blackwood's Edinburgh Magazine, 1891.

2   McCormick pp 77-78.

3   Woodham Smith p376.

4   Carlow Sentinel, 12th August 1848.

5   McCormick p79.

6   McCormick p146.

7   McCormick p80.

8   Carlow Sentinel, 27th May 1848.

CHAPTER 7

1   McCormick p86.

2   ibid.

3   ibid pp 85-86.

4   ibid p88.

5   Arthur Kavanagh Journal of a Tour of India, 1849, (wrongly dated 1858) including Russia and Persia.   KP N6316 P7157.

6   ibid.

7   ibid.

8   Arthur Kavanagh to Lady Harriet Kavanagh, letters 1st June to 5th October 1849. KP N6316 P7156.

9   Wilson, Life and Times of Queen Victoria, Vol 1 p407.

10 Carlow Sentinel, 4th August 1849.

11 ibid. 11th August 1849.

12 Longford, Victoria RI, p191.

13 Arthur Kavanagh to Miss Harriet Kavanagh. KP 1845-51 N6316 P7157.

14 Miss Harriet Kavanagh ibid.

15 Arthur Kavanagh, Nijni Novgorod September 1849. KP   N6316 P7157.

16 McCormick p97.

CHAPTER 8

1   Arthur Kavanagh, Journal of a Tour of India, 10th October 1849.

2   ibid. 11th October 1849.

3   ibid. 12th October 1849.

4   ibid. 10th October 1849.

5   McCormick p102.

6   Arthur Kavanagh, Journal of a Tour of India, 16th November 1849.

7   ibid. 25th December 1849.

8   McCormick p109.

9   McCormick p109.

10 Arthur Kavanagh, Journal of a Tour of India,
    2nd January 1850.

11 ibid. 24th January 1850.

12 McCormick p106.

13 McCormick p121.

14 Cruise of the RYS Eva pp171-3.

15 Arthur Kavanagh, Journal of a Tour of India,
    undated 1850.

16 ibid. undated 1850.

17 Lady Harriet Kavanagh Albanian Journal, 2-15 June 1850.
    KP N6316 P7157.

18 ibid.

19 ibid.

20 McCormick p127.

CHAPTER 9

1   Arthur Kavanagh, Journal of a Tour of India,
    1st & 15th January 1851.

2   ibid. 20th January 1851.

3   McCormick p130.

4   Arthur Kavanagh, 20th January 1851.

5   McCormick p133.

6   Arthur Kavanagh, 21st February 1851.

7   Tom Kavanagh to Lady Harriet Kavanagh.
    KP (letters 1845-51) N6316   P7157.

8   Arthur Kavanagh, 21st April 1851.

9   ibid. undated.

10 McCormick p131.

11 McCormick p132.

12 Steele p140.

13 McCormick p135.

14 ibid. p135.

15 ibid. p140.

16 ibid. p141.

17 Lady Harriet Kavanagh to Tom Kavanagh, 28th June 1852,
    Miscellaneous letters, Borris House.

18 Carlow Sentinel, 21st August 1852.

19 ibid.

20 ibid. 26th February 1853.

CHAPTER 10

1   Carlow Sentinel, 10th February 1849.

2   ibid. 27th January 1849.

3   O'Connel, Carlow Sentinel, 7th January 1837.

4   Mary Dundan O'Leary, Letter of The Rev Sean O'Leary,
    25th April 1986.

5   Carlow Sentinel, 18th June 1854.

6   ibid. 30th December 1854.

7   McCormick p149.

8   Carlow Sentinel, 31st March 1855.

9   ibid.

10 McCormick p149.

11 Carlow Sentinel, 1st September 1855.

12 ibid. 19th January 1850.

CHAPTER 11

1   Arthur Kavanagh Diary, 4th February 1857.
    KP N6315 P7156.

2   ibid. 6th February 1857.

3   Arthur Kavanagh to Frances Kavanagh, Steele pp153-4.

4   Carlow Sentinel, 4th April 1857.

5   Arthur Kavanagh, 2nd April

6   ibid. 27th August

7   ibid. 24th November

8   McCormick p56.

9   Wynne, Fifty Irish Painters NGI.

10 Irish Family Treasures.

11 Arthur Kavanagh, 3rd January 1857.

CHAPTER 12

1 Arthur Kavanagh Diary, 3rd January 1858.

2 ibid. 4th January 1858.

3 ibid. 5th January 1858.

4 ibid. 21st April 1858.

5 Carlow Sentinel, 23rd October 1858.

6 Arthur Kavanagh, 23rd April 1858.

7 ibid. 22nd May 1858.

8 ibid. 22nd July 1858.

9 Carlow Sentinel, obituary of Sir Philip Crampton, July 1858.

10 Wilson, Vol. 2 p22.

11 Arthur Kavanagh Diary, 3rd September 1858.

12 ibid. 19th December 1858.

13 ibid. 8th May 1857.

14 ibid. 6th and 10th January 1859.

15 ibid. 25th December 1858.

16 Arthur Kavanagh 1859 Diary, introductory pages.

17 ibid. 1st January 1859.

18 ibid. 4th January 1859.

19 ibid. 20th February 1859.

CHAPTER 13

1 Arthur Kavanagh Diary, 3rd January 1860.

2 Steele   p129.

3 Arthur Kavanagh Diary, 6th January 1860.

4 ibid. 18th January 1860.

5 ibid. 10th February 1860.

6 ibid. 2nd March 1860.

7 ibid. 6th March 1860.

8 ibid. 25th March 1860.

9 ibid. 22nd April & 22nd June 1860.

10 ibid. 10th April 1860.

11 ibid. 21st April 1860.

12 ibid. 22nd July 1860.

13   The Cruise of RYS Eva, p2.

14   ibid. p50.

15   ibid. p52.

16   Steele p140.

17   Steele pp143,4.

18   RYS Eva p170.

19   McCormick p102

20   ibid. p175.

21   Steele pp132,133.

CHAPTER 14

1   Steele p163.

2   RYS Eva pp1,2.

3 ibid. pp12,13.

4   ibid. p13.

5   ibid. p36.

6   ibid. p47.

7   ibid. pp92,93.

8   RYS Eva p94.

9   ibid. pp109-112.

10   Steele p161.

11   ibid. p141.

12   ibid. p142.

13   Arthur Kavanagh to Frances Kavanagh, 8th June 1864
      Miscellaneous correspondence 1850-70. KP N6316 P7157.

14   ibid. 12th June 1864.

15   ibid. 14th June 1864.

16   McCormick p177.

CHAPTER 15

1   Blackwood's Edinburgh Magazine, 1891.

2   Carlow Post, 21st May 1870.

3   ibid.

4   ibid.

5   Carlow Sentinel, 6th January 1868.

6 Parliamentary Papers, House of Commons,
   Poor Law (Ireland) Amendment Bill, 7th April 1869.

7 ibid.

8 Steele p182.

9 ibid. p175.

10 Parliamentary Papers, House of Commons,
   Union Rating (Ireland) Bill, 20th February 1873.

11 ibid. Irish Land Bill, 1870.

12 Wexford People, 9th July 1870.

13 Parliamentary Debates, House of Commons,
   Land Tenure (Ireland) Bill, 6th February 1878.

14 Parliamentary Papers, House of Commons,
   Land Tenure (Ireland) Bill, 6th February 1878.

CHAPTER 16

1 Parliamentary Debates, House of Commons,
   Ireland - The Press, 17th March 1870.

2 ibid. Peace Preservation (Ireland) Bill,
   22nd March 1870.

3 ibid. Land Tenure Bill (Ireland), 29th June 1876.

4 ibid. Mr Butt's Motion, 30th June 1876.

5 ibid.

6 ibid.

7 Parliamentary Debates, The Municipal Franchise
   (Ireland) Amendment Bill, 6th February 1878.

8 Parliamentary Debates, The University Education
   (Ireland) Bill, 15th May 1879.

9 Wilson, Vol.II p590.

10 Carlow Sentinel, 13th October 1877.

11 ibid.

12 ibid.

13 ibid.

CHAPTER 17

1 McCormick pp185-6.

2 John O'Leary manuscript. CCL.

3 ibid.

4   Carlow Sentinel, 27th March 1880.

5   ibid.

6   John O'Leary manuscript.   CCL.

7   ibid.

8   Blackwood's Edinburgh Magazine, 1891.

9   Arthur McMurrough Kavanagh, 11th April 1880. KP.

10   Report of the Bessborough Commission, 4th January 1881

11   Kee, Robert   p120.

12   Report of the Bessborough Commission.

13   ibid.

14   Gladstone Papers. BL Vol LXXIII   44158.

15   Parliamentary Debates, Land Law (Ireland) Bill,
     7th April 1881.

16   Gladstone Papers. BL Vol CCCLXXXIV 44469 (75).

17   Lieutenant Arthur Kavanagh RN to Lady Harriet
     Kavanagh, undated. KP 6317 P7158.

18   Lieutenant Arthur Kavanagh RN undated.
     KP N3617 P7158.

19   Arthur Kavanagh.   KP N317 P7158.

20   ibid.

21   Arthur Kavanagh to Lady Harriet Kavanagh.
     KP N6317 P7158.

22   ibid.

CHAPTER 18

1   Arthur Kavanagh, The Two Irelands, Steele pp231-244.

2   Steele   p203.

3   Lady Rosebury to W E Gladstone, Gladstone
     Papers, BL Vol. CCCCX 44495, 26th February 1866.

4   Arthur Kavanagh, Gladstone Papers ibid.

5   Steele pp261-262.

6   Steele p262.

7   Carlow Sentinel, 24th July 1885.

8   Steele pp136,137.

9   O'Leary manuscript.

10   Arthur Kavanagh Diary, 31st March 1889.

11   ibid. 9th March 1889.

12   ibid. 31st August 1889.

13   Arthur Kavanagh, Death Certificate, 25th December 1889. GRO.

14   Carlow Sentinel, 4th January 1890.

15   O'Leary manuscript.

16   Carlow Sentinel, 4th January 1890.

IMMEDIATE ANCESTORS AND FAMILY OF ARTHUR MACMURROUGH KAVANAGH

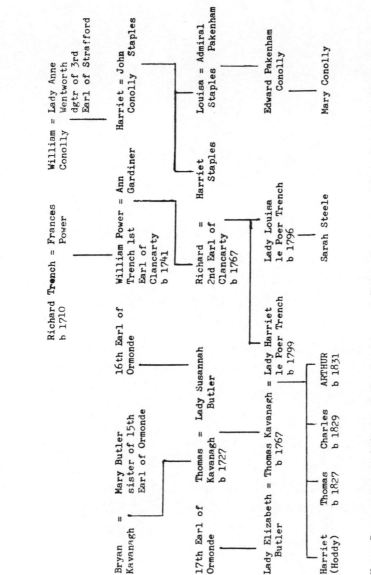

Henry Bruen snr. married one of the daughters of Thomas Kavanagh and Lady Elizabeth Butler. Henry Bruen jnr. married Mary Conolly